Statistics in Toxicology Using R

Ludwig A. Hothorn

Institut für Biostatistik, Leibniz Universität

Hannover, Germany

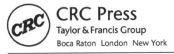
CRC Press
Taylor & Francis Group
Boca Raton London New York

CRC Press is an imprint of the
Taylor & Francis Group, an **informa** business

A CHAPMAN & HALL BOOK

Chapman & Hall/CRC
The R Series

Series Editors

John M. Chambers
Department of Statistics
Stanford University
Stanford, California, USA

Torsten Hothorn
Division of Biostatistics
University of Zurich
Switzerland

Duncan Temple Lang
Department of Statistics
University of California, Davis
Davis, California, USA

Hadley Wickham
RStudio
Boston, Massachusetts, USA

Aims and Scope

This book series reflects the recent rapid growth in the development and application of R, the programming language and software environment for statistical computing and graphics. R is now widely used in academic research, education, and industry. It is constantly growing, with new versions of the core software released regularly and more than 7,000 packages available. It is difficult for the documentation to keep pace with the expansion of the software, and this vital book series provides a forum for the publication of books covering many aspects of the development and application of R.

The scope of the series is wide, covering three main threads:
- Applications of R to specific disciplines such as biology, epidemiology, genetics, engineering, finance, and the social sciences.
- Using R for the study of topics of statistical methodology, such as linear and mixed modeling, time series, Bayesian methods, and missing data.
- The development of R, including programming, building packages, and graphics.

The books will appeal to programmers and developers of R software, as well as applied statisticians and data analysts in many fields. The books will feature detailed worked examples and R code fully integrated into the text, ensuring their usefulness to researchers, practitioners and students.

Published Titles

Stated Preference Methods Using R, *Hideo Aizaki, Tomoaki Nakatani, and Kazuo Sato*

Using R for Numerical Analysis in Science and Engineering, *Victor A. Bloomfield*

Event History Analysis with R, *Göran Broström*

Computational Actuarial Science with R, *Arthur Charpentier*

Statistical Computing in C++ and R, *Randall L. Eubank and Ana Kupresanin*

Basics of Matrix Algebra for Statistics with R, *Nick Fieller*

Reproducible Research with R and RStudio, Second Edition, *Christopher Gandrud*

R and MATLAB® *David E. Hiebeler*

Statistics in Toxicology Using R *Ludwig A. Hothorn*

Nonparametric Statistical Methods Using R, *John Kloke and Joseph McKean*

Displaying Time Series, Spatial, and Space-Time Data with R, *Oscar Perpiñán Lamigueiro*

Programming Graphical User Interfaces with R, *Michael F. Lawrence and John Verzani*

Analyzing Sensory Data with R, *Sébastien Lê and Theirry Worch*

Parallel Computing for Data Science: With Examples in R, C++ and CUDA, *Norman Matloff*

Analyzing Baseball Data with R, *Max Marchi and Jim Albert*

Growth Curve Analysis and Visualization Using R, *Daniel Mirman*

R Graphics, Second Edition, *Paul Murrell*

Introductory Fisheries Analyses with R, *Derek H. Ogle*

Data Science in R: A Case Studies Approach to Computational Reasoning and Problem Solving, *Deborah Nolan and Duncan Temple Lang*

Multiple Factor Analysis by Example Using R, *Jérôme Pagès*

Customer and Business Analytics: Applied Data Mining for Business Decision Making Using R, *Daniel S. Putler and Robert E. Krider*

Implementing Reproducible Research, *Victoria Stodden, Friedrich Leisch, and Roger D. Peng*

Graphical Data Analysis with R, *Antony Unwin*

Using R for Introductory Statistics, Second Edition, *John Verzani*

Advanced R, *Hadley Wickham*

Dynamic Documents with R and knitr, Second Edition, *Yihui Xie*

CRC Press
Taylor & Francis Group
6000 Broken Sound Parkway NW, Suite 300
Boca Raton, FL 33487-2742

First issued in paperback 2021

Version Date: 20151116

ISBN 13: 978-1-03-209813-5 (pbk)
ISBN 13: 978-1-4987-0127-3 (hbk)

Publisher's Note
The publisher has gone to great lengths to ensure the quality of this reprint but points out that some imperfections in the original copies may be apparent.

Visit the Taylor & Francis Web site at
http://www.taylorandfrancis.com

and the CRC Press Web site at
http://www.crcpress.com

Contents

9   Conclusions   **205**

Appendix: R Details   **207**

References   **209**

Index   **233**

List of Figures

List of Tables

Preface

When you write a book on *statistics in toxicology* you are sitting on the fence: For statisticians much is known (or at least not exciting), but a large number of toxicologists will be overwhelmed. This book was prepared with a minimum of mathematical formulas, but on the basis of real data examples that are explicitly evaluated with specific R programs. Hence, the second part of the title "*Using R*" was selected.

The book is primarily structured according to selected toxicological assays, and, based on statistical methods. This style comes at the price of somewhat annoying repetitions and many cross-references.

The book is available in print. However, in addition there is a `knitr` [409] document and the package "*SiTuR*", which on the notebook under R can run all data examples by definition. This provides an additional way of learning: Replacing selected data examples through your own data.

Looking at current toxicological publications closely, notice that the core problem *is a significant test of a criterion for hazard*—or perhaps more important: *is non-significance a criterion for harmlessness*—is not really solved. The apparent contradiction between statistical significance and biological relevance has greatly reduced the importance of statistics in decision making—thus reducing the value of statistical methods as a whole in toxicology. One aim of this book is to highlight ways out of this dilemma.

Following the establishment of regulatory toxicology in the 1970s, many statistical methods for toxicology have been published. Regardless, the recommendations for statistical analysis remain remarkably imprecise in most toxicological guidelines; even the pinnacle, the experimental design, remains imprecise. The second aim of this book is to present assay-specific proposals, e.g., for the *in vitro* micronucleus assay. It provides suggestions, not recommendations, and is certainly not a cookbook!

The statistical complexity varies substantially in this book: From the *t*-test to the mixing distribution approach in the Comet assay trying to describe the appropriate evaluation.

The statistical analysis of experimental data is a current standard in toxicology. In almost every paper, statistical methods are used. Tests and their *p*-values are dominating today—explicitly or at least implicitly for claiming significant effects. Toxicology is a broad field. This book focuses on standardized bioassays for chemicals (by OECD guidelines, e.g., [283]), drugs (by ICH guidelines, e.g., [199]) and environmental pollutants (by EPA, OECD and ECOTEC guidelines [12, 282]) and consequently hypothesis testing is the focus. Accordingly, the book is organized initially by selected bioassays: i) short-term repeated toxicity studies, ii) long-term carcinogenicity assays, iii) studies on reproductive toxicity, iv) mutagenicity assays, and v) toxicokinetic studies. Methodically oriented chapters follow: vi) proof of safety, vii) toxicogenomics, viii) toxicokinetics, ix) analysis of interlaboratory studies and x) modeling of dose–response relationships for risk assessment.

For some readers, this text will appear testing heavy. Yes, it is. Six arguments speak in favor of hypothesis testing against modeling: i) the only focus in the related US National

Toxicology Program (NTP) recommendation [9], ii) the main focus of most guidelines, iii) commonly used designs with two or three doses only (+ zero dose control), iv) availability of dose metameters only–probably not simply related to the concentrations at the target in the bioassays nor to the human exposure, v) superiority of modeling only when very specific assumptions hold true and vi) the preferred method in recent publications in experimental toxicology.

The challenge was a representation style using few formulas for sometimes complex statistical methods. The first focus is on raw *data*, *data* structures, and *data* models. The second focus is **using R packages**. The third focus is reproducible publication [191] by means of a single `knitr` document containing all the raw data, R code, text, figures, tables, statistical outcomes, references. That is, educationally the following order is adhered to: a brief explanation of the toxicological problem, followed by the equally short explanation of the statistics, the matching data example (structure, raw data, visualization), the R code, the outcomes and their interpretation.

This allows a toxicologist to select a certain bioassay, e.g., the Ames assay, to understand the specific data structure (counts, small samples, non-monotone dose-response effect etc.), to run the R code with the data example, understand the test outcome and the interpretation, and replace the data set with his/her own data and run again.

All data that are used in this book are either available in the package `SiTuR` or otherwise in cited R packages.

To the reader I want to apologize for the less than perfect figures and tables; my focus was direct processability in `knitr`, i.e., to achieve a reproducible document.

Acknowledgments

Without the cooperation of the following colleagues, this book would not have been possible: G. Dilba Djira (Brookings), G. Gerhard (Christchurch), M. Hasler (Kiel), E. Herberich (Ingelheim), T. Hothorn (Zurich), Th. Jaki (Lancaster), A. Kitsche (Hannover), F. Konietschke (Dallas), R. Kuiper (Utrecht), P. Pallmann (Lancaster), Ch. Ritz (Copenhagen), F. Schaarschmidt (Hannover), and Z. Zhkedy (Hassel) —this is particularly true for making available the R packages `multcomp`, `mratios`, `pairwiseCI`, `MCPAN`, `ETC`, `goric`, `drc`, `bmd`, `statint`, `toxbox`, `Isogene`, `coin`, `nparcomp`, `PK`. Also, I would like to acknowledge the free availability of numerous raw data by the US NTP database (`http://ntp.niehs.nih.gov/results/dbsearch/index.html`).

Moreover, I thank L. Edler (Heidelberg), A. Kopp-Schneider (Heidelberg), R. Pirow (Berlin), C. Vogel (Hannover) and A. Krueger (Braunschweig) for the critical comments when reading draft chapters.

I am grateful to three anonymous reviewers for the constructive and encouraging comments which improved the quality substantially.

1

Principles

1.1 Evaluation of short-term repeated toxicity studies

The principles of design and evaluation are discussed in the following by means of selected items in short-term repeated toxicity studies. The aim of repeated dose toxicity studies is to characterize the toxicological profile of a compound usually administered between 4 weeks [283] and 3 months [284]. Although baseline values or data of a recovery period are available in some studies, the typical data are multiple endpoints at the end of the administration period, such as continuous endpoints (e.g., hemoglobin), rates (e.g., proportions of histopathological findings), or ordered categorical data (e.g., graded histopathological findings). The standard design uses a negative control (C) and several doses $D_1, ..., D_k$ where $k = 3$ is common. A one-way layout will be considered during evaluation, i.e., both sexes are analyzed independently (see their joint analysis in Section 2.4.1) The comparisons of doses versus control are performed by unadjusted two-sample tests (see Section 1.3), or the Dunnett procedure [102] without order restriction (see Section 2.1.1) or the Williams procedure [400] with order restriction (see Section 2.1.2). The usual sample sizes per group i, $n_i = 10$ in rodent studies allow the use of standard tests, including asymptotic ones, though only under particular assumptions, or only for selected endpoints. For all other endpoints and particularly small sample sizes like in dog studies, specific tests are needed. This small sample size restriction is the first feature of statistics in toxicology; it is repeatedly discussed in the book.

> Features:
> - Principle of statistical inference in toxicology
> - Proof of hazard without control of the familywise error rate (FWER)
> - Two sample comparisons for continuous, skewed variables, proportions and counts

1.2 Selected statistical problems

1.2.1 Data visualization by barcharts or boxplots?

Up to now the most common style of data presentation are tables containing group-specific means, standard deviations, and sample sizes, commonly for multiple endpoints; see e.g.,

[376] in Figure 1.1.

Table 1 Effect of tBOOH on cellular integrity, redox status, and Ca^{2+} levels

	DMSO[a]	tBOOH[b]
Cellular viability (% of total cells)	96 ± 3	$62 \pm 3*$
LDH release (% of total cell content)	32 ± 2	$42 \pm 3*$
ATP cellular content (μmol/10^6 cells)	48 ± 6	43 ± 3
MDA cellular content/nmol/mg prot.)	1.3 ± 0.2	$8.0 \pm 0.3*$
Total glutathione (mg/mg of protein)	27 ± 2	$17 \pm 1*$
GSSG-to-total glutathione ratio (%)	3.1 ± 0.1	$4.1 \pm 0.2*$
Cytosolic free Ca^{2+} (nM)	119 ± 11	$3029 \pm 474*$

Cells were pretreated for 15 min either with tBOOH (500 μM) or with DMSO (controls)

LDH lactate dehydrogenase, *ATP* adenosine triphosphate, *MDA* malondialdehyde, *GSSG* oxidized glutathione

* $p < 0.05$ versus DMSO, for $n = 4$–10

FIGURE 1.1: Example for data summary table.

Bar charts are commonly used as well, e.g., [98] used barcharts (including SEM) and letters of significance (Figure 1.2).

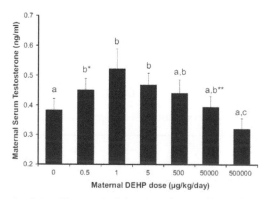

Fig. 2. Effect of different doses of DEHP on maternal serum testosterone concentrations on GD 18 (ANOVA on log-transformed data, $P < 0.05$). Values represent the mean $\pm$ SEM. Treatments with the same letter are not significantly different from each other but are statistically different from groups with other letters. b*, $P = 0.07$ relative to controls; b**, $P = 0.09$ relative to 500,000 group. Sample sizes were: oil $n = 20$; 0.5 μg, $n = 9$; 1 μg, $n = 11$; 5 μg, $n = 12$; 500 μg, $n = 13$; 50 mg, $n = 16$; 500 mg, $n = 17$.

FIGURE 1.2: Example of bar charts.

Although both representations allow a dense display, they have two major drawbacks: they assume normally distributed data (and we know how often this is violated in real data) and they do not allow access to the individual data. Individual datapoints have a special meaning in toxicology, because sometimes the relevant information is contained just in a few extreme values —not necessarily in means. Therefore, Rhodes et al. [319] visualized just group-specific individual data (by dots) for 20 rats together with the (geometric) mean (in Figure 1.3):

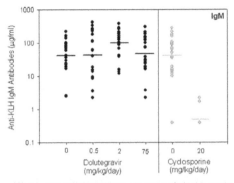

FIG. 2.   IgM anti-KLH TDAR in juvenile rats treated with dolutegravir. Sera were harvested 5 days post-KLH immunization and assessed for anti-KLH IgM antibodies by quantitative electrochemiluminescent immunoassay. Circles represent individual animals (n = 20/group) with geometric mean indicated by the bars. There were no detectable dolutegravir-related effects on the anti-KLH IgM antibody response when juvenile animals received daily treatment. In rats given the positive control for immunosuppression (20 mg/kg/day of cyclosporine), there was a significant decrease (p < 0.001) in the level of anti-KLH IgM antibodies. Eighteen of 20 rats given 20 mg/kg/day of cyclosporine tested below the IgM assay lower limit of quantification and were assigned a value of 0.4 µg/ml for the purpose of calculating group geometric mean.

FIGURE 1.3: Example of individual data representation.

Surprisingly, boxplots are rarely used in toxicology (see e.g., [75] in Figure 1.4), although, they were recently recommended in a points-to-consider paper [108].

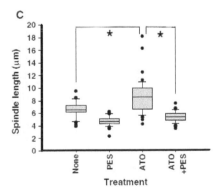

FIGURE 1.4: Example for boxplot in toxicology.

A boxplot typically uses nonparametric measures of location and scale, namely median and interquartile range ($IQR = q_{0.75} - q_{0.25}$) as well as an outlier rule (represented by whiskers), e.g., $k * IQR; k = 1.5$ (notice, $q_{0.75}$ is the 75% percentile). The boxplot provides simple information on group-specific location, variance, and asymmetry of distribution as well as existence of extreme values. Outlier identification or even elimination is rather critical in safety assessment (see Section 2.5) and this k-rule should not be used without specific care [357]. For grouped data a specific jittered boxplot was developed in the R `library(toxbox)` (see details [294]) which provides: i) nonparametric measures median, IQR, ii) parametric measures mean and standard deviation, iii) individual data, iv) graphic differentiation between randomized unit and technical replicates (e.g., pregnant rats and pups), v) sample sizes, and vi) signs of significances. The inappropriateness of barcharts compared to jittered boxplots (available in the package `toxbox`) is demonstrated by litter-specific pup weight data [390] in Figure 1.5 (see further details in Section 5.2).

```
> data("ratpup", package="WWGbook")
> Ratpup <-ratpup
> Ratpup$Treatment <-factor(Ratpup$treatment,
+    levels=c("Control","Low","High"))
> Ratpup$litter <- as.factor(Ratpup$litter)
```

This specific version of boxplots is used throughout this book for grouped data; here is the R-code:

```
> library("toxbox")
> boxclust(data=Ratpup, outcome="weight", treatment="Treatment",
+ cluster="litter", ylabel="Pup weights in g", xlabel="Dose",
+ option="dotplot", vline="fg", hjitter=0.01, legpos="none", printN=TRUE,
+ white=TRUE, titlesize=8, labelsize=6)
> data.raw <-ratpup
> data.raw$value <-data.raw$weight
> data.summary <- data.frame(
+    treatment=levels(data.raw$treatment),
+    mean=tapply(data.raw$value, data.raw$treatment, mean),
+    n=tapply(data.raw$value, data.raw$treatment, length),
+    sd=tapply(data.raw$value, data.raw$treatment, sd)
+ )
> data.summary$treat <-factor(data.summary$treatment,
+                      levels=c("Control","Low","High"))
> library("ggplot2")
> ggplot(data.summary, aes(x = treat, y = mean)) +
+    geom_bar(position = position_dodge(), stat="identity", fill="gray") +
+    geom_errorbar(aes(ymin=mean, ymax=mean+sd)) +
+    ylab("Pup weights in g") +
+    xlab("Treatment") +
+    ggtitle("Bar plot with standard deviation as error bars.") +
+    theme_bw() +
+    theme(panel.grid.major = element_blank())
```

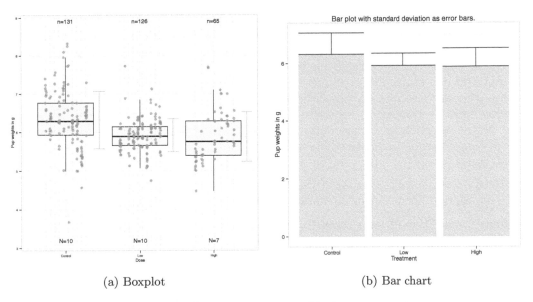

(a) Boxplot   (b) Bar chart

FIGURE 1.5: Comparing two graphical representations.

The bar chart visualizes just means and standard deviations (SD) (assuming normal distribution), whereas in the boxplots the raw data, parametric and nonparametric summary measures (namely means, standard deviation; median, interquartile range), the individual data (dots), and the per-litter structure (including group-specific number of litters and the number of plots) can be seen. For incidences or graded histopathological findings mosaic plots can be used for visualization; see e.g., Section 2.1.8.

1.2.2 How to present tests' outcomes: Stars, letters, p-values, or confidence intervals?

Four different presentation styles of statistical tests can be found in the literature: i) rejection/non-rejection of H_0 (where letters indicate non-distinguishable treatment groups; see an example below), ii) rejection of H_0 for three α levels (0.05, 0.01, 0.001) visualized by stars $*, **, * * *$, iii) p-value (p), and iv) confidence interval. Stars are still common when results of chronic toxicity studies are presented; see e.g., [119] for selected hematological endpoints. A p-value is a near-to-zero skewed probability, reflecting the falsification principle: *we can never prove an effect directly, only demonstrate how unlikely its opposite is*. The p-value is a measure of this unlikeliness as a probability between $[0, 1]$ [100]. A confidence interval provides the possible range of a particular effect size (such as $\mu_i - \mu_C$ or μ_i/μ_C), for example, 95% of future data (where μ_i is the expected value in group i). The width of the confidence interval is a measure for the uncertainty, depending on variance(s), sample size(s), the false positive decision probability, and possibly other aspects of the assumed statistical model and test procedure. It contains information on: i) the rejection/non-rejection of H_0 by inclusion/non-inclusion of the value of H_0 (i.e., 0 for difference and 1 for ratio), ii) the interpretation of biological relevance by the distance of the confidence limit(s) to this value of H_0 in terms of the measured unit (difference) or percentage change (ratio), and iii) the directional decision (i.e., whether increasing or decreasing effects occur). Therefore, confidence intervals should be preferred [99, 26], particularly their consistent use for both proof of safety and proof of hazard [28]. In the ICH E9 guideline [198] their use is recommended for the evaluation and interpretation of randomized clinical trials; a related recommendation for toxicological studies is still missing. Today the most common presentation style in this field is the p-value due to its simplicity. Due to its smallness, the distance to H_0 in terms of a probability characterizes the magnitude of statistical significance. Summarizing, this book focuses on test decisions primarily by means of confidence intervals, and secondarily by compatible tests and their p-values. Therefore, the primary criterion should be the selection of an adequate effect size, namely for the difference of expected values $\mu_i - \mu_0$, the ratio μ_i/μ_0, the difference of proportions $\pi_i - \pi_0$, the ratio of proportions (relative risk) π_i/π_0, the odds ratio of proportions $\frac{\pi_i/(1-\pi_i)}{\pi_0/(1-\pi_0)}$, and the relative effect size $p_{i0} = Pr(X_i < X_0) + \frac{1}{2}Pr(X_i = X_0)$ (where X_i is a value in group i) (see details in Section 2.1.4)—appropriate for toxicological reasoning for a particular endpoint.

The joint visualization of data characteristics and statistical significances is a challenge. Here, different styles are demonstrated using an example of triglycerides in clinical chemistry for a control and three doses in a 13-week study with sodium dichromate dihydrate to F344 rats [16]. The raw data are presented in Table 1.1.

```
> data("clin", package="SiTuR")
```

Table 1.1: Raw Data of Serum Triglyceride of a 13-Week Study

Dose	Triglyceride
0	236.00
0	102.00
0	144.00
0	130.00
0	125.00
0	93.00
0	235.00
0	67.00
0	145.00
...	...
1000	85.00
1000	80.00
1000	29.00
1000	55.00
1000	59.00
1000	32.00
1000	79.00
1000	70.00

A possible visualization is a factorplot [32] which contains all-pair comparison adjusted p-values with the estimates and errors in a matrix. Because such a matrix is helpful when considering many all-pairs comparisons it is not demonstrated here.

Multiple plots are preferred, with Figure 1.0a containing on the left side jittered boxplots and on the right side simultaneous confidence intervals for Dunnett-contrasts using the package `multcomp` (Figure 1.6b). A sometimes used visualization style is a letter plot for distinguishable treatment groups together with boxplots [304]. The package `multcompview` is a realization for all-pair comparisons whereas, in Figure 1.7a, the function `cld` (compact letter display) in the package `multcomp` is used for any multiple contrasts. Notice,

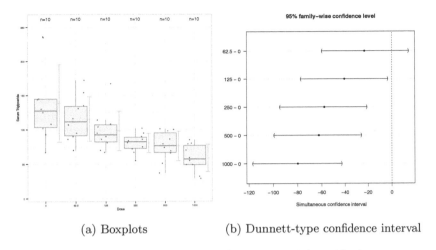

(a) Boxplots (b) Dunnett-type confidence interval

FIGURE 1.6: Multiple plots for serum triglyceride data.

throughout the book 95% confidence intervals are used and if not not will be stated clearly. Alternatively on the right side, a combination of boxplots with Dunnett-type p-values (Figure 1.7b) (or in the form of stars; see e.g., Section 1.2.2) [294] is displayed. This style allows for a maximum of interpretation.

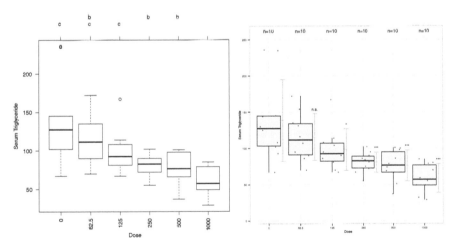

(a) Letter-type representation of signifi- (b) Boxplots with Dunnett-type stars
cances

FIGURE 1.7: Two plots with signs of significance for serum triglyceride data.

1.2.3 Proof of hazard or proof of safety?

The main objective of a study in regulatory toxicology is to decide whether a new drug entity or chemical is harmless, harmless up to a specified dose, or harmful. The final determination regarding the harmlessness or harmfulness is a complex process where much more is needed than just statistical tests.

1.2.3.1   Decision making in toxicology

First, the p-value of a statistical test is widely used in decision making: a finding is classified as positive when $p < 0.05$ or negative when $p > 0.05$. As an example, the criteria for positive response in the OECD 486 guideline for the UDS assay (unscheduled DNA synthesis) is defined as " *NNG (net nuclear grain) values significantly greater than concurrent control*" [289]. However, common statistical tests are formulated for a point-zero null hypothesis, such as the t-test, Wilcoxon–test, or χ^2-test, i.e., each tiny non-relevant change versus control can be significant, for example, in the case of small variances. Conversely, large effect sizes can be deemed "not significant" simply because the sample size was too small for the inherent variability of the particular endpoint.

Second, a modified decision rule is used that takes the magnitude of the spontaneous tumor rate into account. The two significance levels for a positive Cochran–Armitage [31] trend test for proportions are: $p < 0.025$ for rare tumors and $p < 0.005$ for common tumors [14]. This rule reflects the specific sensitivity of tests on proportions depending on the spontaneous proportion.

Third, trend tests are used for claiming a positive trend because the common designs in toxicological assays include a negative control and several doses. For example, in the OECD 479 guideline for the *in vitro* sister chromatid exchange assay (SCE) a criterion is formulated as: "*... statistically significant dose-related increase in the mean number of SCEs per cell*" [11].

Fourth, relevance thresholds are used, e.g., in the local lymph node assay (LLNA) a positive response is concluded when the stimulation index is larger than 3 [286]. Most relevance criteria are formulated for relative change, such as the k-fold rule in the Ames assay [70], and therefore inference relative to control is needed. However, these relevance thresholds ignore the assay's uncertainty. Here, the estimation of confidence intervals for ratio-to-control comparisons is proposed, where their estimated limits are used *posthoc* to interpret relevant (proof of hazard; see Sections 1.3, 2.1) or tolerable change (proof of safety; see Section 2.5).

1.2.3.2   Be confident in negative results

Due to the falsification principle of Neyman–Pearson tests, two concepts should be distinguished: i) the proof of hazard, i.e., demonstrating harmfulness and ii) the proof of safety, i.e., demonstrating harmlessness. In the first approach the probability of erroneously concluding hazard, i.e., producer's risk (false positive error rate), will be controlled directly. In the second approach the probability of erroneously concluding safety, i.e., consumer's risk (false negative error rate $f-$) is controlled directly [58, 262]. (Notice, alternatively the term power is used, whereas power is simply $1 - f-$.) For drug safety assessment, the consumer's risk seems to be more important, along the lines of: "*be confident in negative results*" [181, 260]. Failing to reject the null hypothesis in the proof of hazard ($p > 0.05$), often leads to the conclusion of evidence in favor of harmlessness. However, it is important to realize: "*absence of evidence is no evidence of absence*" [27, 28]; this can lead to problematic decisions. Therefore, both the widely used proof of hazard and the rarely used proof of safety are described in the following; see particularly Sections 2.1 and 2.5.

1.2.3.3 Several two-sample comparisons or multiple comparisons versus control?

For the common design, which includes a control and several doses, the US National Toxicology Program (NTP) [9] recommends analysis by the Dunnett procedure [102] and/or Williams procedure [400]. These proof of hazard approaches control the familywise error rate (FWER). The term *familywise* is a bit difficult to understand —*family* consists exactly of the k comparisons against control for k dose or treatment groups. A more appropriate term is *claimwise error rate* [301], where *claim* consists of the identification of at least one up to k doses/treatments different to control. Therefore, Dunnett/Williams procedure is rather conservative compared to independent level α-tests (see Section 1.3). Commonly, a significant dose-related trend test is used as causation criteria, e.g., in [290] *"...there are several criterion for determining a positive result, such as a concentration-related increase...".* The commonly used test for comparing doses versus control under the assumption of monotonicity is the Williams procedure [400]. Therefore, this procedure is the main approach in this book and modifications used for the different endpoint types occurring in toxicology will be provided, e.g., for proportions, counts, poly-3 counts, survival functions, and ranks. Evaluating an efficacy endpoint in a clinical dose finding study by Dunnett's procedure is appropriate because the claim of a particular effective dose, a related α penalty should be paid. In contrast, within toxicology the aim is not to select a certain toxic dose and therefore the control of the comparisonwise error rate (CWER) seems to be sufficient. For this purpose, k independent two-sample comparisons $Cvs.D_i$, each at level α, are described in Section 1.3. This approach is used in order to achieve lower false negative rates (which is equivalent to higher power) compared to approaches controlling FWER. In order to show the difference between FWER and CWER, a fictional example containing the comparison of 3 doses vs. control is given based on the Bonferroni inequality (FWER control) in comparison to independent t-tests (CWER control) $(n_i = 20, \sigma/\delta = 1,$ two-sided t-tests)$(\sigma$ ... root of variance, δ ... difference to be detected). The main differences are the elementary α levels of $\alpha^{CWER} = 0.05$, and a much smaller $\alpha_i^{FWER} = 0.05/3 = 0.01666$. Both false negative decision rates can be simply calculated:

```
> fnC <-1-power.t.test(n =20, delta =1, sd = 1, sig.level = 0.05)$power
> fnF <-1-power.t.test(n =20, delta =1, sd = 1, sig.level = 0.01667)$power
```

Consequently, the *posthoc* false negative error rates for the CWER approach of 0.131 is much smaller than those of the FWER approach (0.258). This illustrates a basic dilemma in toxicology caused by applications of Dunnett-type evaluation in most reports and publications. (Please notice, that throughout this book the correlation between test statistics is used, therefore all FWER-approaches, such as Dunnett test, are less conservative than the Bonferroni approach which is only used here to keep the example simple.)

For a particular toxicological assay, statistical significance or biological relevance is rarely explicitly defined. The second part of the OECD recommendation [290] focuses on biological relevance, i.e., *"...a reproducible increase in the number of cells containing micronuclei".* Therefore, related simultaneous confidence intervals will be described primarily. For some assays, adjusted p-values will be reported in order to achieve adaptability to common publication style (dominated by p-values). In the following, two types of proof of hazard are discussed: without and with control of FWER. In Section 1.3 independent two-sample comparisons will be discussed, whilst in Section 2.1 the Dunnett- and Williams-type procedures for multiple comparisons versus control will be discussed. The main focus here is the Williams procedure for several types of endpoints. Simultaneous confidence intervals, allowing a claim for relevance, are of primary interest.

1.2.4   Sample size matters

In most guidelines the minimum required sample size for a toxicological assay is specified, e.g., at least triplicate plates in the Ames assay [287] or at least 5 animals per sex in the micronuclei assay (MN) [288]. For point-zero hypotheses in the proof of hazard, the secondary error rate (false negative rate f^-) is therefore endpoint-specific, depending on the variance, the common $\alpha = 0.05$ level and several assumptions such as Gaussian distribution. Still, the minimum required sample sizes ensure a certain standardization of the false negative rate ($power = 1 - f^-$) and should be used in practice. In the proof of safety, the secondary error rate depends additionally on the endpoint-specific tolerance threshold θ_i (see Section 2.5). Another aspect regarding relatively small sample sizes, such as triplicated plates in the Ames assay, is the specific finite properties of the tests. For example, asymptotic non-parametric tests do not control level α approaches, whereas permutation tests are rather conservative. Furthermore, the impact of variance heterogeneity is serious in both tests because both assume variance homogeneity.

Therefore, the small sample size behavior of the tests and procedures is considered in this book, as a specific feature of inference; see e.g., [46].

Outside of regulatory toxicology, sample sizes are sometimes chosen arbitrarily, i.e., not statistically planned in advance. The limitation of interpreting p-values becomes obvious, since the p-value is a direct function of sample size. In order to illustrate this, we generate simulated datasets containing the same expected values (means), and the same variances, but (balanced) sample sizes 5, 10, and 15.

```
> library(SimComp)
> set.seed(17059101); muC=7.6; muT=9.3; sC=1.54; sT=1.72
> exp5C <- ermvnorm(n=5,mean=muC,sd=sC)
> exp5T <- ermvnorm(n=5,mean=muT,sd=sT)
> exp10C <- ermvnorm(n=10,mean=muC,sd=sC)
> exp10T <- ermvnorm(n=10,mean=muT,sd=sT)
> exp15C <- ermvnorm(n=15,mean=muC,sd=sC)
> exp15T <- ermvnorm(n=15,mean=muT,sd=sT)
> endpoint5 <-c(exp5C, exp5T)
> factor5 <- factor(rep(c("Control", "Treatment"),c(5,5)))
> dat5 <- data.frame(endpoint5,factor5)
> endpoint10 <-c(exp10C, exp10T)
> factor10 <- factor(rep(c("Control", "Treatment"),c(10,10)))
> dat10 <- data.frame(endpoint10,factor10)
> endpoint15 <-c(exp15C, exp15T)
> factor15 <- factor(rep(c("Control", "Treatment"),c(15,15)))
> dat15 <- data.frame(endpoint15,factor15)
> p5 <-round(t.test(endpoint5~factor5, data=dat5)$p.value,3)
> p10 <-round(t.test(endpoint10~factor10, data=dat10)$p.value,3)
> p15 <-round(t.test(endpoint15~factor15, data=dat15)$p.value,3)
```

The Welch-t-test p-value for the small-sample size study is 0.139, for medium-sample size 0.032 and for larger-sample sizes 0.008. This example should warn against over-interpretation of p-values in unplanned studies.

A p-value depends, of course, primarily on the effect size, but also directly on the sample size (as well as the variance and other items such as the validity of the distribution assumption). The p-value has a predictive value in toxicological decision making in planned studies (*a priori* assuming a minimum effect size) or at studies using guideline-recommended n_i, but not for studies where n_i results from non-statistical reasons such as feasibility.

1.2.5 Multiplicity occurs

For Phase III clinical trials the adjustment against several sources of multiplicity (multiple endpoints, multi-regional trials, subgroups, repeated studies) is essential [42, 301]. Thus, the concept of a claimwise error rate was proposed [301] which is more realistic than FWER. In safety assessment multiplicity-adjustment should be used with care due to its conservativeness. The standard design in toxicological studies includes a negative control and some doses: $C, D_1, ..., D_k$, and therefore the US National Toxicology Program proposed Dunnett [102] and/or Williams [400] tests [9], both controlling FWER. Moreover, multiple endpoints, such as multiple tumor sites occur and the question arises whether and how multiplicity adjustment should be performed. A quite different approach is used for the proof of hazard or the proof of safety. Both union-intersection (i.e., *OR* links between multiple hypotheses) and intersection-union hypotheses (i.e., *AND* links between multiple hypotheses) will be discussed. Along with this, several methods for multiplicity adjustment are discussed in this book.

1.2.6 Several types of endpoints occur

A contradiction may exist in toxicology. Whereas most publications on statistics in toxicology focus on continuous endpoints, such as organ weights, the most relevant information is contained in counts and proportions, such as tumor rates or graded histopathological findings, for which only few statistical approaches exist. Three main types of endpoints can be distinguished: i) vital signs, e.g., number of offspring per live female in *Ceriodaphnia dubia* assay [249], ii) pathological findings, e.g., number of micronuclei in the MN assay [176], and iii) physiological parameters, e.g., serum bilirubin concentration [19]. Endpoints measured by vital signs are used in inhibition assays, which are particularly suitable for ratio-to-control tests on non-inferiority, since their continuous variable, or count, or proportion decreases from large values in the control (sometimes 100%) to small values in the dose groups, i.e., the reduction of offspring is a sign of toxicity. In the second group, the data in the control are often zero or near-to-zero, requiring specific tests. For the third type of endpoints, increases or decreases may be of toxicological interest.

Several types of endpoints occur, e.g., continuous normal and non-normal variables, proportions, mortality-adjusted tumor rates, graded findings, counts, time-to-event data; and therefore corresponding endpoint-specific tests are discussed in this book.

1.2.7 Directional decisions

Although a controversy on the appropriateness of one-sided tests exists (see, e.g., [245]), one-sided tests for the first two categories of endpoints ((i.e., inhibition/non-inferiority endpoints and near-to-zero endpoints)) are clearly suggested. For both endpoints the opposite direction can be toxicologically irrelevant. For example, in a carcinogenicity study only increasing tumor rates are of interest; possibly decreasing tumor rates are toxicologically irrelevant. Moreover, one-sided hypotheses are inherently needed for non-inferiority tests (see Section 2.5.1). Furthermore, one-sided tests or confidence limits should be preferred to limit the false negative error rate and are plausible for dose-related trend tests. Even for the third category of endpoints, a directional decision after a significant two-sided test is needed (which is closed under intersection) because not only a significant change but also its direction is of interest. Hereby, the control of the directional error rate is of particular interest, that is the rate for a decision in the false direction [122]. Please notice, appropriate one-sided tests and confidence intervals for differences of proportions for small sample sizes between $n_i = 10$ (90-days study) and about $n_i = 50$ (long-term carcinogenicity study) are a challenge. Due to their conservativeness, exact approaches, such as the exact Fisher test or permutation Wilcoxon–test, should be avoided in toxicology (see further discussions [248, 259]). Thus, approximate one-sided confidence intervals are provided for comparing treatments versus control, trend evaluation, and claiming non-inferiority. Please notice, related confidence intervals for ratio-to-control or odds ratio are unstable for near to zero spontaneous rates and should be avoided. Therefore, in this book one-sided confidence intervals (and their compatible tests) are of particular interest.

1.2.8 Specific designs

The common completely randomized design is $[C, D_{low}, D_{med}, D_{high}]$. Rarely, more or less dose groups are included. Balanced designs are recommended, i.e., the same sample size in each group. However, due to the power optimality rule of the Dunnett procedure, special unbalanced designs were proposed, i.e., using $\sqrt{k}$ higher sample size in the control. Notice, this rule remains valid only under variance homogeneity [93]. Further design issues are dual controls and positive controls. Dual controls should be avoided, as they are not required by guidelines, make variance heterogeneity more serious, and increase total sample size. Positive controls are highly recommended, first to guarantee assay sensitivity (by demonstrating a substantial effect size versus negative control), and second to demonstrate non-inferiority of dose effects relative to the positive control [37]. Unfortunately, the use of a selected positive control with a certain concentration is not common in toxicology. If both sexes are used, as in rodent studies, they are commonly evaluated independently (which is conditionally a conservative approach). Particularly, for large animals such as dogs and primates, the sexes are analyzed together to compensate for the rather small sample sizes. In some studies more complex layouts occur, including blocks (e.g., cages), a secondary factor (e.g., sex), hierarchical sub-units (e.g., pup weight within a female), technical replicates (e.g., 50 cells per gel and animal in the Comet assay), repeated measures (e.g., body weight curves), and covariates (e.g., body weight in organ weight analysis). Commonly simplified solutions are used (such as relative organ weights instead of covariance analysis), or per condition analysis is preferred (such as separate per-sex analysis) or block effects are ignored. Additionally, related appropriate approaches are available, focusing on the primary comparison of dose groups versus control, e.g., for repeated measures.

Therefore, the specification of a design with doses and a zero-dose control is primarily discussed in the book, extended for secondary fixed factors, sub-units, technical replicates, blocks, repeated measures, and covariates; see Section 2.4.

1.2.9 Mixing distribution and outliers

Most statistical textbooks assume unimodal distributions, though not necessarily normal. Nevertheless, the tolerance model of toxicology, in which *the affected population consists of τ responders and $(1 - \tau)$ non-responders* would lead to a mixing distribution, that is not a unimodal distribution. However, a bimodal (or even a k-modal) distribution may exist, consisting of an unknown proportion $(1 - \tau)$ of animals behaving similarly to control animals and τ responding animals. Inference for mixing distributions exists, e.g., [170], but the common small sample size makes these approaches complicated (see Section 2.1.10). However a large number of sub-units occur in toxicology, such as scored cells or comet length for many cells in gel electrophoresis. Here, specific mixing distribution approaches can be used; see Section 4.12. Particularly, for small sample sizes it can happen that just one reacting animal cannot be distinguished from an outlier. Therefore, formal statistical tests on outliers should generally be avoided in toxicology (particularly in connection with their removal); a further reason is that the underlying distribution is unknown.

1.2.10 The phenomenon of conflicting decisions

In each animal several endpoints are measured or surveyed in repeated dose toxicity studies. Some are continuous, such as body weight, some are proportions, such as histopathological incidences, and some are ordered categorical, such as graded histopathological findings. For all these endpoints the decision is based on the same maximum false positive rate $\alpha = 0.05$ and the same sample sizes n_i. The detectable effects for an equal assumed false negative rate of say $\beta = 0.20$ are therefore extremely different. For example, we assume the body weight in $n_i = 10$ control rats is about 420 g and the standard deviation SD=14 g. For the one-sided t-test the detectable effect difference to a dose group is about 16 g. For a proportion with a spontaneous response rate of 0%, only an incidence difference to 45% in any dose group can be detected. For graded findings with 90% in category 0, 5% in category +, 2.5% in category ++ and +++ in the control, a shift to 40% in category 0, 20% in category +, 25% in category ++ and 15% in category +++ can only be detected [224]. This means that the same detection sensitivity is found: i) for an increase of 3.3% body weight, ii) for an increase of incidence from 0 to 45%, and iii) for a shift from 90% to 40% in category 0. This example characterizes the basic contradiction: small differences of precise measured continuous endpoints, which may have a low toxicological importance, can be detected. In contrast, only well-pronounced differences for either incidence rates or graded findings, which may have a high toxicological importance, can be detected.

Therefore, in this book appropriate and robust procedures for normal, continuous, proportions endpoints and counts are discussed and, in particular, their small sample behavior is discussed.

1.2.11 Decision tree approaches

One of the myths in applied biostatistics is that in the case of heterogeneous variances, the Wilcoxon–test (for two samples) or the Steel-type test (for comparing treatments vs. control, i.e., a nonparametric version of the Dunnett test) are robust, whereas, the t-test (or the Dunnett test) is not robust. For example in the method section of [407] it is explicitly written: *"...when the variance was heterogeneous based on Bartlett's test, the Steel's multiple comparison test was employed."* Therefore, decision tree approaches, consisting of a pre-test on variance homogeneity (to be precise: on variance heterogeneity) or other conditions, such as normal distribution, followed by the optimal selected main test, are quite common. Three major arguments exist against this conditional two-step approach, the so-called decision tree approach:

i) the conditional two-step approach does not control level α [419]: *"...preliminary tests of equality of variances used before a test of location are no longer widely recommended by statisticians, although they persist in some textbooks and software packages. The present study extends the findings of previous studies and provides further reasons for discontinuing the use of preliminary tests "*,

ii) nonparametric tests or procedures are inappropriate for heterogeneous variances [418]: *"...the Student t test maintains its significance level more consistently than the Wilcoxon–Mann–Whitney test when variances of treatment groups are unequal and sample sizes are equal,"*
iii) conditional tests are problematic [154]: *"...many books on statistical methods advocate a conditional decision rule when comparing two independent group means. This rule states that the decision as to whether to use a pooled variance test that assumes equality of variance or a separate variance Welch t test that does not should be based on the outcome of a variance equality test. Several unconditional tests including the separate variance test performed as well as or better than the conditional decision rule... conditional decision rule should be abandoned. "*

Moreover, even for normal distributed variables, for unbalanced designs and variance heterogeneity, the Steel-type procedure tends to be conservative when high variances occur at large sample size and to liberal behavior (i.e., FWER is not controlled when high variances occur at small sample size). In the simulation study [271], for a design using $n_i = 35, 25, 20, 15$ and $SD_i = 1, 3, 3, 3$ the empirical FWER is 0.098 for the Steel procedure whereas for the parametric counterpart (Dunnett) it is 0.060; i.e., the decision tree assumption is seriously violated. Ruxton (2006) [329] recommended the Welch-t-test as an alternative to both the t-test and the Mann–Whitney U test. A further decision-tree problem is the use of a global ANOVA conditional or unconditional before the Dunnett procedure (or in the nonparametric setup the Kruskal–Wallis global test before the Dunn or Steel procedure), as described in the US NTP documents [9]. This is inappropriate for several reasons: i) from the view of the closed testing procedure after a significant F-test, level α t-tests "control vs. doses" form a closed intersection hypotheses system; it is not the procedure itself controlling the FWER. Performing the Dunnett procedure only after a significant F-test is an unnecessarily conservative approach, which should be avoided in toxicology [183], ii) the alternative regions of the F-test and the Dunnett procedure are different; the first is defined for an all-pairs alternative, the second for a simple tree alternative; and iii) the F-test is a quadratic form whereas the Dunnett test is a linear form as a special case of multiple contrast tests; see Section 2.1.1.1.2. Therefore, the F-test should not be used in a one-way layout at all. Rarely two- or higher-way layouts are used in toxicology (e.g., sex or time as a secondary factor), and here the F-test is used for testing interactions *a priori*. But even here, interaction contrast is a more appropriate technique [348]; see Section 2.4.1.

Therefore, in this book decision tree approaches are not proposed.

1.2.12   The special importance of control groups

Assays without a negative control group are unthinkable in toxicology. Therefore inference versus the concurrent negative control is the dominating approach; see Sections 1.3 and 2.1. Multiple similar assays allow the use of the information of their historical controls, either directly into the test decision (in Section 4.10) or the estimation of reference values (in Section 2.3). Positive controls are less common, but can be used either for claiming assay sensitivity or for demonstrating the relevance of a change versus negative control by using a non-inferiority test (in Section 4.11).

Therefore, procedures for comparisons against the negative control $(C-)$, procedures for comparisons against the positive control $(C+)$, and the use of historical control group information will be discussed in this book.

The preferable design includes both a negative control, some dose groups and a positive control. It allows simultaneous decisions on superiority against $C-$ and non-inferiority against $C+$ (see details in Section 4.11).

As an example, micronucleus data with the treatment groups `Vehicle`, `Hydro30`, `Hydro50`, `Hydro75`, `Hydro100`,`Cyclo25` were selected [152] (see details in Section 4.11).

```
> data("Mutagenicity", package="mratios")
> Muta <- Mutagenicity
> Muta$Treatment <- factor(Muta$Treatment, levels=c("Vehicle","Hydro30",
+                          "Hydro50", "Hydro75","Hydro100","Cyclo25"))

> library("mratios")
> MutaP <-droplevels(Muta[Muta$Treatment !="Vehicle", ])
> pposs <-simtest.ratioVH(MN~Treatment, data=MutaP,
+                   alternative="less", type = "Dunnett", base = 5,
+                   Margin.vec=c(0.8,0.8,0.8,0.8))$p.value.adj
> MutaN <-droplevels(Muta[Muta$Treatment !="Cyclo25", ])
> pnegs <-simtest.ratioVH(MN~Treatment, data=MutaN,
+         alternative="greater", type = "Dunnett", base = 1)$p.value.adj
> MutaPN <-droplevels(Muta[Muta$Treatment %in% c("Vehicle", "Cyclo25"), ])
> ppn <-t.test.ratio(MN~Treatment, data=MutaPN, alternative="less")$p.value
```

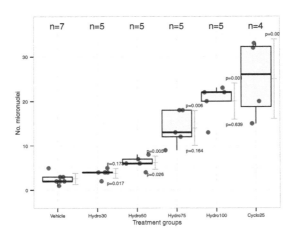

FIGURE 1.8: Micronucleus data including a positive control.

Figure 1.8 shows the jittered boxplots with adjusted p-values for Dunnett-type ratio-to-control comparisons: the lower for comparisons against $C-$, the upper for comparisons against $C+$. MNs in the Hydro100 dose are substantially increased against $C-$ (p-value

0.001) and 80% non-inferior to $C+$ (p-value 0.639). The p-value for the positive control stems from claiming assay sensitivity by a t-test for the two-sample problem $[C-, C+]$.

In some bioassays dual controls are used, commonly water and solvent control. The primary aim seems to be the identification of a possible specific effect of the solvent. This cán be easily tested by two-sample tests described in Section 1.3. In many cases these controls do not really differ [132] and the possibility of pooling exists to increase control sample size and hence the power of the tests against control [131]. A pre-test is recommended to test for no serious difference between both controls. An equivalence test can be used; see Section 2.5. But the choice of the equivalence thresholds remains an open problem.

1.2.13   Statistical significance and biological relevance

A not uncommon practice in toxicology is to interpret selected significant findings as biologically not relevant. A less common, but more important, practice is to interpret insignificant findings as relevant. This contradiction between significance and relevance has several reasons, among them the use of tests for a point-zero null hypothesis. For example, for the UDS assay in the OECD 486 guideline *"...NNG values significantly greater than concurrent control"* are defined as positive outcomes. Confidence intervals should be used ([99, 279]) and interpreted with respect to an *a priori* defined relevance threshold, denoted as the minimal clinically important difference [208], e.g., 100 ml for lung function through FEV_1 (an expiratory volume parameter). Using a toy example, five outcome types can be distinguished, as can be seen in Figure 1.9 for a simulated dataset:

- Statistically not significant D1-NC

- Significant without clinical relevance D2-NC

- Not significantly less than threshold D3-NC

- Probably clinically significant effect D4-NC

- Large clinically significant effect D5-NC

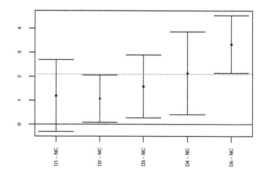

FIGURE 1.9: Simulated data for different patterns of significance and relevance.

From a toxicological point of view, the scenario *probably clinically significant effect* (D4-NC) is of particular interest, i.e., the effect size (here mean difference) is above the relevance threshold (i.e., certain biological relevance) and the lower confidence limit larger than zero (i.e., formal statistical significant). For this scenario the sample size can be estimated [212]. For example, for an assumed effect difference $\delta = 3.0$, a standard deviation of $\sqrt{\sigma^2} = 2.3$, a false positive rate $\alpha = 0.05$, and a false negative rate $\beta = 0.2$, a sample size for the point-zero hypothesis (i.e., scenario of just statistical significance D2-NC) of $n_i = 8$ is needed (two-sided t-test with balanced sample sizes). For a scenario of significance and relevance (i.e., probably clinically significant effect (D4-NC)), a sample size of $n_i = 10$ is needed where the point estimator must be at least 2.1 (dotted line in Figure 1.9). These sample size estimations can be performed by the package WinProb using the concept of win probabilities [155].

A further argument for relevance is not only to consider a significant dose-response relationship for a particular endpoint in a single study, but also to consider a similar effect for multiple endpoints. Examples are negligible bias due to maternal toxicity in developmental studies, different dose-response patterns for different endpoints (e.g., malformations at low doses but fetal death at higher doses), taking into account cluster effects (i.e., a single malformation in 10 litters is not the same as 10 malformed pups in a single litter), similar effects for multiple studies and different species and supportive arguments from quite different mechanisms (e.g., toxicokinetics); see the rare definition of levels of evidence in developmental toxicology [117].

1.3 Proof of hazard using two-sample comparisons

1.3.1 Normal distributed continuous endpoints

In principle, the common two-sample tests, such as the t- or Wilcoxon–test, each at level α can be used here. As an example selected clinical chemistry data from the 13-week study with sodium dichromate dihydrate to F344 rats [16] is used; see part of the raw data in Table 1.2. In a data.frame format for a factor Dose and several endpoints (blood urea nitrogen (BUN), serum creatinin (Creat), albumin (ALB), serum glucose (SerumGlucose), creatine kinase (CreatKinase), anilin aminotransferase (ALT)) for each animal (i.e., row) complete values exist.

```
> data("clin", package="SiTuR")

> library("pairwiseCI")
> welcht <-pairwiseCI(value ~ dose, data=mclin, by="variable",
+        method="Param.diff", var.equal=FALSE, control="0")
> plot(welcht, lines=c(1,0.5, 2),  lty=c(1,2,2), CIcex=0.5,
+      cex.axis=0.28, cex.main=0.15, main=NULL)
```

Confidence intervals for Welch-t-tests can be used assuming normal distribution and allowing heterogeneous variances. However, they are scale-specific which makes a comparative interpretation complicated; see Figure 1.10. Therefore, this subsection focuses on confidence intervals for ratio-to-control comparisons in order to allow claiming biological relevance (vs. statistical significance) over differently scaled multiple endpoints. Here the effect size is percentage change which is dimensionless. Two-sample one-sided or two-sided confidence intervals for the ratio to control according to Fieller [116] are available modified in the case of variance heterogeneity [367]. These intervals allow scale-independent interpretation, which

Table 1.2: Clinical Chemistry Raw Data of Sodium Dichromate Bioassay

Dose	BUN	TP	ALB	SerumGlucose	CreatKinase	ALT
0	17.3	7.4	5.0	137.0	202.0	100.0
0	15.0	6.9	4.7	180.0	205.0	56.0
0	15.7	7.1	4.9	164.0	188.0	70.0
0	16.5	7.1	4.9	145.0	155.0	54.0
0	16.7	7.2	5.0	126.0	160.0	64.0
...	...	...	...	...	...	...
1000	17.4	5.7	4.0	142.0	444.0	182.0
1000	17.4	6.2	4.3	125.0	401.0	118.0
1000	18.7	6.1	4.2	141.0	337.0	222.0
1000	20.5	6.1	4.2	146.0	838.0	322.0
1000	19.0	6.7	4.7	113.0	370.0	288.0

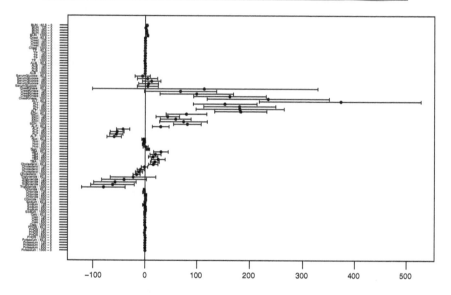

FIGURE 1.10: Welch-*t*-test confidence limits for clinical chemistry endpoints.

is particularly helpful for multiple endpoints in hematology and clinical chemistry. Naturally, this approach is limited to data containing control values different from zero, where variances and sample sizes are taken into account. By means of the R package `pairwiseCI` for all clinical chemistry endpoints, related dose-specific confidence intervals can be easily estimated. The numeric variable `Dose` should be transformed into the factor `Dose` and the row-wise structured multiple endpoints should be transformed into a secondary factor `variable` by the function `melt`. These two-sided confidence intervals for ratio-to-control comparisons allowing variance heterogeneity, independent of each endpoint and each dose, are presented in Figure 1.11. The related R-code is simple:

```
> library("pairwiseCI")
> tratio <-pairwiseCI(value ~ dose, data=mclin, by="variable",
+         method="Param.ratio", var.equal=FALSE, control="0")
> plot(tratio, H0line=c(1,0.5, 2),  H0lty=c(1,2,2), CIcex=0.5,
cex.axis=0.29, main=NULL)
```

We see that confidence limits of most endpoints and most comparisons are within a range between [0.5; 2], but some endpoints, such as ALT, reveal a strong and statistically signif-

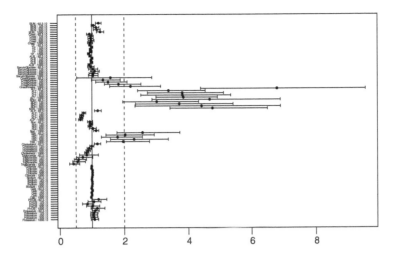

FIGURE 1.11: Ratio-to-control confidence intervals for clinical chemistry endpoints.

icant increase. The task of the toxicologist is to interpret these significant increases and to determine if they are toxicologically relevant,particularly in the context of all available findings. Please notice, this plot is suitable for screening non-normal findings because of its rather liberal behavior due to only comparison-wise error control between multiple doses and between multiple endpoints.

Alternatively, related *p*-values or confidence intervals for the differences to control can be estimated easily using the R package `pairwiseCI` using the option `method="Param.diff"` (see Figure 1.10).

1.3.2 Log-normal distributed continuous endpoints

A usual approach for the often skewed biological data is to apply a log-transformation. The back-transformed confidence intervals of the t-test represent as an effect size the ratio of medians which are hard to interpret. A more appropriate approach for log-normal distributed endpoints is available [74]. Even more extreme conditional tests based on data transformation are used in toxicology as a third alternative, i.e., [85] *"...if Bartlett's test was not significant at the 1% level, then parametric analysis was applied. If Bartlett's test was significant at the 1% level then logarithmic and square-root transformations were performed and if Bartlett's test was still significant, then nonparametric tests were applied."* Such an approach cannot be recommended; see the arguments in the decision tree Section (1.2.11).

Related confidence intervals can be estimated using the parameter `methods="Lognorm .ratio"` in the package `pairwiseCI` [338]:

```
> library("pairwiseCI")
> par(mar=c(4,8,3,1))
> lognorm <-pairwiseCI(value ~ dose, data=mclin, by="variable",
+       method="Lognorm.ratio", var.equal=FALSE, control="0")
> plot(lognorm, H0line=c(1,0.5, 2),  H0lty=c(1,2,2), CIcex=0.5,
+ xlab="Ratios-to-control for log-normal endpoints",cex.axis=0.29,main=NULL)
```

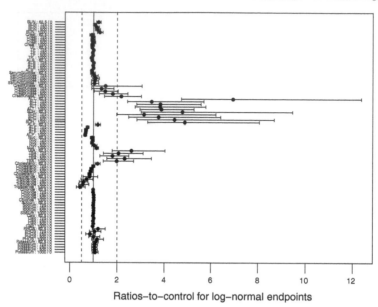

Ratios–to–control for log–normal endpoints

FIGURE 1.12: Confidence limits for log-normal distribution.

1.3.3 Non-normal distributed continuous endpoints

The common approach for endpoints with a skewed distribution and/or extreme values is the Wilcoxon–test. Sometimes a Behrens–Fisher problem occurs, i.e., the two groups differ primarily according to their locations but heterogeneous variances occur as well. Please notice, the Wilcoxon rank sum test is not suitable for variance heterogeneity, particularly in unbalanced designs [210]. There is a common related misuse; see e.g., evaluation of the chronic toxicity study on 1,3-dichloropropene [362]. Alternatives, such as the asymptotic rank-transformed Welch-t-test [420] cannot be recommended because simulations reveal inflated α levels [89] which are similar to their bootstrap modification [317] and to their α inflation under heteroscedasticity [378]. Despite its common use, data transformation to achieve variance homogeneity, (e.g., log transformation), is dangerous because transformation of the data prior to testing necessarily changes the null hypothesis under test [402]. Furthermore, the median test cannot be recommended because of its low power [65]. Adaptive tests consisting of several tests for several alternatives [278] are not recommended here because their alternative is not clearly defined and hence its toxicological interpretation is problematic and confidence intervals are not available. A particular alternative is the asymptotic nonparametric Behrens–Fisher test [62]. However, this test does not control the α level for small sample sizes and therefore modifications were introduced: a t-distributed version [62] and a permutation version [277]. By using the relative effect size [62], the null hypothesis $H_0 : p = \frac{1}{2}$ can be tested for two independent random variables X_1 and X_2 with any distributions F_1 and F_2 to: $p_{12} = Pr(X_1 < X_2) + \frac{1}{2}Pr(X_1 = X_2) = \int F_1 dF_2$. That is, p_{12} represents the probability that a randomly chosen subject in treatment group 1 reveals a smaller response value X_1 than a randomly chosen subject from treatment group 2 with response value X_2. If $p < 1/2$, then the values in group 1 tend to be larger than those in group 2. If $p = 1/2$, none of the observations tend to be smaller or larger. In the special case of independent ordinal data, p_{12} is called the ordinal effect size [331, 330]. Parametric tests use as effect size the difference (or ratio) of means, but for biomedical trials an effect size on an individual basis is of interest [61], such as the relative effect size. In summary, all these arguments for and against nonparametric tests in comparison to parametric tests make the decision for one or the other complicated, this is true especially in small sample designs [29]. Nonparametric intervals for the difference to ratio according to [163] and for ratio to control [271] can be used. The related confidence intervals can be estimated using the parameter `methods="HL.ratio"` (where HL stands for Hogdes–Lehmann [163], specific nonparametric estimates):

```
> library("pairwiseCI")
> mclin0 <-droplevels(mclin[mclin$variable!="Creat", ])
> HLL <-pairwiseCI(value ~ dose, data=mclin0, by="variable",
+                  method="HL.ratio", control="0")
> mclin0 <-droplevels(mclin[mclin$variable!="Creat", ])
> par(mar=c(4,8,3,1))
> plot(HLL, H0line=c(1,0.5, 2),  H0lty=c(1,2,2),  CIcex=0.3,
+ xlab="Nonparametric ratio-to-control comparisons",
+ cex.axis=0.22, main=NULL)
```

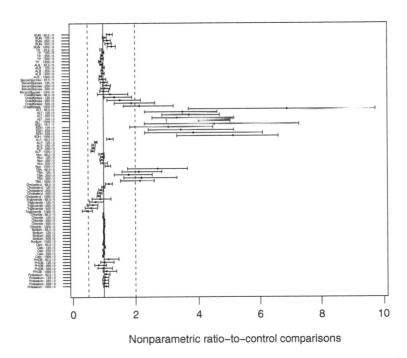

Nonparametric ratio–to–control comparisons

FIGURE 1.13: Nonparametric confidence limits for clinical chemistry endpoints.

1.3.4 Proportions

Up to now, an almost confusing number of publications on confidence intervals (and tests) for proportions in 2-by-2 tables (e.g., [257]) exists. Even with these, tests or confidence intervals for proportions in both 2-sample and k-sample designs are still a challenge. In toxicology for the analysis of crude mortality, findings or animal specific MN/PCE proportions (MN/PCE ...number of micronuclei per scored polychromatic erythrocytes), etc. rather specific conditions occur:

- Extremely small samples sizes (see 1.2.10). (Notice, $n_i = 10$ is *small* for the asymptotic Wilcoxon–test, but *extremely small* for a test on proportions)

- Both two-sided and one-sided hypotheses are of interest. However, switching from two-sided to one-sided intervals is not as simple as switching the quantile in t-test intervals $t_{df,1-\alpha/2} \Rightarrow t_{df,1-\alpha}$. One-sided limits may not provide a valid level $\alpha/2$ decision in situations where the two-sided intervals provide a level α decision. Even the approaches for lower limits, needed in the proof of hazard, and for upper limits, needed in the proof of safety, are not always the same [340].

- Zero or near-to-zero proportions in the control may happen, particularly for pathological responses such as tumor incidences. This data condition may cause serious problems when using a GLM-approach (see for details Section 2.1.5.1)

- Three different effect sizes for the expected proportions $\pi_i = Y_i/n_i$ are available and are used, though are not necessarily appropriate (where Y_i is the absolute number of effects). Although the risk difference $(\pi_i - \pi_0)$ is dominating in toxicology, the risk ratio (π_i/π_0) and the odds ratio $(\frac{\pi_i/(1-\pi_i)}{\pi_0/(1-\pi_0)})$ can be used as well. Actually, the choice of effect measure should depend on the design and interpretability, but it depends also on the data conditions and the numerical stability of the estimates. Risk ratio approaches are unstable when either the control rate is zero or the treatment rate is near to one and therefore should be used with care.

- Proportions occur on the level of the treatment factor, e.g., number of tumors in the high dose (with respect to number at risk), or on the level of each individual animal, e.g., animal-specific MN/PCE. In the first case, the 2-by-2, or 2-by-k table data can be analyzed, in the second case the variability between the animals should be modeled: either by estimation of the overdispersion (see Section 2.1.5.4) or by a mixed effect model with the random factor animal (see Section 2.1.5.4.1)

- Modified proportions occur, e.g., the poly-3 estimates by mortality-adjustment of tumor incidences (see 3.5)

- Stratified tables exist, e.g., for the analysis of incidental tumors (see Section 3.4.1)

- Tests and confidence intervals are not necessarily compatible

Although widely used, Fisher's exact test can be too conservative for small sample sizes [83], a contraindication for toxicology. On the other hand, approximate Wald-type intervals may seriously violate the coverage probability of 95%, particularly in case of near-to-zero control data. Therefore, the use of approximations can be suggested where *adding one pseudo-observation to success and to failure* [22] (denoted as ADD-2 approach), i.e., the Wald-type proportion $p_i = Y_i/n_i$ is replaced by $\tilde{p}_i = (Y_i + 1)/(n_i + 2)$. This is simple and efficient for risk differences [346] and for odds ratios [234] to control the coverage probability approximately. Please notice, for one-sided lower limits even adding one pseudo-observation, i.e., $\tilde{p}_i^{one-sided} = (Y_i + 0.5)/(n_i + 1)$ is appropriate [340, 346]. These interval estimates are numerically available in the R package `pairwiseCI` [341]. As an example histopathological tubular epithelia findings in the P-Cresidine carcinogenicity study [201] are used here, where 2-by-2 table data were selected (see Table 1.3).

Table 1.3: 2-by-2 Table Data for Tubular Epithelia Findings

Groups	Without	With
Control	10	0
High	2	8

```
> data("tubepi", package="SiTuR")
> tub2 <-droplevels(tubepi[tubepi$Group %in% c("Control", "High"),])

> library("pairwiseCI")
> tubOR <- pairwiseCI(cbind(TubularEpithelia,Without) ~ Group, data=tub2,
+                     alternative="greater", method="Prop.or",
+                     CImethod="Woolf", control="Control")
> tubD <-pairwiseCI(cbind(TubularEpithelia,Without) ~ Group, data=tub2,
+                     alternative="greater", method="Prop.diff",
+                     CImethod="AC", control="Control")
> tubRR <-pairwiseCI(cbind(TubularEpithelia,Without) ~ Group, data=tub2,
+                     alternative="greater", method="Prop.ratio",
+                     CImethod="MOVER", control="Control")
```

The difference of proportion is 0.8 where a significant increase with a magnitude of 0.423 in terms of the difference of proportions (95% lower limit) can be stated. The ratio of proportions cannot be estimated. The odds ratio is 71.4 where a significant increase with a magnitude of 5 in terms of an odds ratio was found.

1.3.5 Counts

Counts do not occur too frequently in systemic toxicology, as graded histopathological findings are common. In contrast, counts are the typical endpoints of *in vivo* or *in vitro* assays, such as number of micronuclei (MN) (see Section 4.6). Counts are also very common in sublethal ecotoxicity data, such as number of *Lemna fronds* or number of offspring for invertebrates. Already mentioned, one-sided testing is appropriate, since only an increase of severity is of interest. Three serious problems occur when comparing two counts of small sample sizes, such as ($n_i = 10, 10$): i) the power is rather small (compared with continuous endpoints), ii) the asymptotic tests for comparing two counts do not control the α level, and iii) the count measured per animal varies within each treatment group, i.e., an excess variability may exist. Related confidence intervals for the ratio of two counts exist by: i) fitting a generalized linear model with family definition of quasi-poisson using the function glm by constructing a deviance profile and deriving an equal-tailed confidence interval from this profile, ii) fitting a generalized linear model with log-link using the function glm.nb in package MASS by constructing a likelihood profile and deriving an equal-tailed confidence interval for the negative binomial model. Both intervals are available in the package pairwiseCI [341].

As an example, the two-sample problem with both a negative and a positive control for the number of micronuclei (Vehicle,Cyclo25) is used (see details in Sections 4.11 and 1.2.12). The related confidence interval can be estimated assuming Poisson-distributed counts with overdispersion between the animals using the parameter methods="Quasipoisson.ratio":

```
> library("pairwiseCI")
```

```
> hyaCI <-pairwiseCI(MN ~ Treatment, data=MutaPN, alternative="greater",
+                       control="Vehicle", method="Quasipoisson.ratio")
> hyaCI3 <-as.data.frame(hyaCI)
```

For this ratio-to-control comparison, the ratio is 9.72 and its lower confidence limit is 5.99, i.e., the number of micronuclei is more than doubled, i.e., this assay is sensitive. Please notice the limited precision of this confidence limit because of the rather small sample sizes.

1.3.6   Further endpoint types

The analysis of multinomial variables (such as differential blood count) (see Section 2.1.7), ordered categorical data (such as graded histopathological findings) (see Section 2.1.8), hazard rates (such as mortality functions) (see Section 3.2.2), transformed endpoints (such a transformed near-to-zero counts) (see Section 4.7), censored time-to-event endpoints (see Section 3.6.4) and multivariate endpoints (see Section 3.6.2) are described in the related chapters in detail.

Simultaneous comparisons of dose or treatment groups against a negative control group is THE dominating approach for both short-term and long-term bioassays. This approach is described in detail in a separate chapter.

2

Simultaneous comparisons versus a negative control

2.1 Proof of hazard using simultaneous comparisons versus a negative control

2.1.1 Normally distributed continuous endpoints: The Dunnett procedure

Without any doubt, the Dunnett procedure is one of the most widely used statistical tests in toxicology: 692 of the 3514 citations of the original paper [102] (WebSci January 2014) are applications in toxicology. Moreover, it is recommended by the US NTP [9]. It belongs to multiple comparison procedures which control the familywise error rate. If the control of the familywise error rate is intended, an increase of the false negative rate has to be accepted. This increase can be restricted by 1) minimizing the number of simultaneous comparisons, e.g., least number of dose groups or avoiding all-pairs comparisons procedures (such as Duncan procedure [326]) ii) using one-sided confidence intervals instead of two-sided, iii) taking correlations between the simultaneous comparisons into account, e.g., using Dunnett's procedure instead of the p-value based step-wise approach according to Holm [167], iv) restricting the alternative due to monotonicity, e.g., using Williams procedure, v) still restricting the alternative even when downturn effects may happen at high doses by means of downturn protected Williams procedure [54, 204], and vi) avoiding designs with higher control sample size (and hence less n_i in the dose groups) when variance heterogeneity may occur, particularly lower variance in the control (on the other hand $n_C >> n_{D_i}$ is recommended when $s_C > s_{D_i}$). Hereafter, a completely randomized one-way layout $[C, D_1, ..., D_k]$ is considered. In Section 2.4 more complex layouts, including blocks (e.g., cages), a secondary factor (e.g., sex), hierarchical sub-units (e.g., pup weight within a female), repeated measures (e.g., body weight curves), and covariates (e.g., body weight in organ weight analysis) will be discussed.

Features:

- Dunnett/Williams-type procedures for almost all occurring endpoint types
- Proof of hazard with control of the familywise error rate (FWER)
- Trend tests
- Analysis of complex designs: Interactions, block designs, covariates, repeated measures
- Proof of safety

2.1.1.1   The Dunnett procedure

The US NTP recommends the evaluation of continuous variables (which revealed approximately normal distributions in historical controls) with the parametric multiple comparison procedures of Dunnett [102]. Up to now it is the standard in published studies in toxicology; see e.g., the preclinical characterization of the abuse potential of methylphenidate [372]. Remarkable is its use for claiming the lack of an effect by reporting non-significant p-values, e.g., concerning the effect of butylparaben and methylparaben on the reproductive system in male rats [162].

Most multiple comparison procedures can be formulated as multiple contrast tests. Several single contrast tests [123, 174, 56, 173] with $T_l = \frac{\sum_{i=0}^{k} c_{li} \bar{X}_i}{S \sqrt{\sum_{i=0}^{k} c_{li}^2 / n_i}}$ $(1 \le l \le k)$ are used in which the definition of the contrast coefficients c_{li} depends on the formulated alternative hypotheses (where S is the root of the common means square error estimator, X_i are the treatment mean value, n_i the sample sizes and i the treatment index, e.g., $i = 0$ for the negative control and $i = 1$ for the lowest dose). For one-sided differences the contrast matrix is:

$$
C = \begin{pmatrix}
-1 & 0 & \dots & 0 & 1 \\
-1 & 0 & \dots & 1 & 0 \\
\vdots & \vdots & \dots & \vdots & \vdots \\
-1 & 1 & \dots & 0 & 0
\end{pmatrix}
\tag{2.1}
$$

The vector $(T_1, \dots, T_k)'$ follows a joint k-variate t-distribution with $df = \sum_{i=0}^{k}(n_i - 1)$ degrees of freedom and a correlation matrix $\mathbf{R} = (\rho_{ij})$ given by

$$
\rho_{ij} = \sqrt{\frac{1}{(1 + n_0/n_i)(1 + n_0/n_j)}} \quad (1 \le i \ne j \le k).
$$

(for the simplified case of homogeneous variances and the use of a common mean square error estimate S). The lower one-sided $(1-\alpha)100\%$ simultaneous confidence limits are given by

$$
\hat{\delta}_i^l = \bar{X}_i - \bar{X}_0 - t_{k,1-\alpha}(df, \mathbf{R}) \, S \sqrt{\frac{1}{n_i} + \frac{1}{n_0}};
$$

Endpoints, whose increase is questionable, can be declared hazardous if the lower limit is relevantly larger than zero. In other words, endpoints with a lower limit above 0 have increased significantly to control and the distance to zero —expressed in the underlying measurement scale —can be used as a criterion of relevance. As an example the endpoint creatine kinase of the clinical chemistry data in a 13-week study [16] was selected; see this part of the raw data in Table 2.1.

```
> data("clin", package="SiTuR")
```

It can be seen in boxplots in Figure 2.1 that creatine kinase increases with increasing doses, variance heterogeneity, and extreme values, such as 1135 in the 62.5 mg/kg dose group.

Before Dunnett-type simultaneous confidence intervals are estimated by means of the function `glht` within the package `multcomp`, the fit of a linear model (for one-way analysis of

Table 2.1: Raw Data of Serum Creatine Kinase in a 13-Week Study

Dose	CreatKinase
0	202
0	205
0	188
0	155
0	160
...	...
1000	444
1000	401
1000	337
1000	838
1000	370

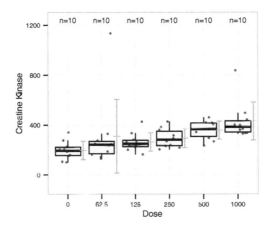

FIGURE 2.1: Boxplots of the clinical data creatine kinase using ordinal dose metameters.

variance assuming normal distributed error and homogeneous variance) is needed, at which the object `mod1` contains all needed estimates. The estimation of simultaneous confidence intervals (two-sided) or limits (one-sided) is quite simple using the function `glht` (*generalized linear hypotheses test*) within the R package `multcomp` where the contrast matrix in eq. 2.1 is simply defined by the argument `"Dunnett"` [189]. If no further arguments are chosen, 95% two-sided confidence intervals are computed by default.

```
> library("multcomp")
> mclinA$Dose <-as.factor(mclinA$Dose)
> mod1 <-lm(CreatKinase~Dose, data=mclinA)
> plot(glht(mod1, linfct = mcp(Dose = "Dunnett")),
+      main="",xlab="Difference to control" )
```

The two-sided confidence intervals for all differences to control (Figure 2.2) indicate a significant increase only for the highest dose. However, because of possible variance heterogeneity, a Welch-type modification should be used for real data analysis; see the related Williams procedure in Section 2.1.2.

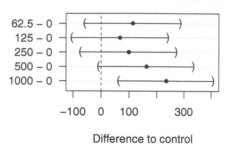

Difference to control

FIGURE 2.2: Dunnett-type simultaneous confidence intervals for serum creatine kinase.

2.1.1.1.1 Robustness

The concept of robustness is highly relevant for non-statistician users, particularly when a test is explicitly proposed in guidelines such as the Dunnett-test. Here the question arises: is this test still appropriate in case the underlying distribution assumption is violated? Sometimes not even all assumptions are explicitly formulated for a particular test at a first glance. Because violations do not follow a black-or-white pattern, robustness will not provide a black-or-white answer but a tendency. Further questions may concern whether the Dunnett/Williams test still can be used in case data reveal non-normality, outliers, heterogeneity of variances, missing values, non-monotonicity (Williams test), and/or extreme small sample sizes (particularly for the modifications for ranks, proportions, Cox-model etc.). On this subject predominantly simulation studies [328, 169, 379, 275] exist. The Dunnett procedure modified for heterogeneous variances is more robust than expected. Particularly, in usual small sample size designs, it is almost the best of all bad options. One general trend can be discerned: toward smaller sample sizes the effect of violating the assumptions becomes more critical (i.e., a too conservative or too liberal false positive rate occur), especially if several assumptions are violated simultaneously (such as skewed distribution and heterogeneous variances). However this is very typical in toxicological studies and therefore the selection of appropriate tests remains critical. Further relevant research would be necessary.

2.1.1.1.2 F-test and Dunnett procedure

Sometimes, the use of Dunnett's test is proposed only after a significant ANOVA F-test. For example the US NTP states: *"...if the ANOVA is significant at $p < 0.05$ or less, Dunnett's multiple range t test is used for multiple treatment-control comparisons"* ([9]) or *"... analyzed by using either parametric or nonparametric analysis of variance followed by contrasts estimating the pairwise differences between each dosed group and vehicle control or by using Williams trend test or Dunnett t-test..."* ([207]). On the other hand, an unconditional approach is used, e.g., dose-response assessment of nephrotoxicity by independent ANOVA and Dunnett's test ([203]). This questions the use of F-test **and** Dunnett procedure. A well-known decision-tree approach is the closed testing procedure [253] in which after a significant F-test pairwise t-tests can be performed, each at level α. This is especially simple for comparisons against control [359], e.g., $F_\alpha^{C,D_1,D_2,D_3} \Rightarrow [t_\alpha^{C,D_1}, t_\alpha^{C,D_2}, t_\alpha^{C,D_2}]$. However, the F-test is followed by pairwise t-tests, not by Dunnett tests. In this case simultaneous confidence intervals are difficult to interpret [50]. A consistent conditional approach would require a strictly larger power of ANOVA F-test than of the Dunnett's test for all possible data conditions in which the global null hypothesis is false. This is not the case, particularly for alternatives of the form $0, \delta, ..., \delta$ in specific unbalanced designs [183]. Stopping after a non-significant F-test, although the Dunnett's test would give at least one significant finding, increases the false negative error, which is problematic in toxicology. A simple example demonstrates this unfortunate behavior. The lung weights (`LungWt`) of female mice after 13 weeks of per os administration of acrylonitrile were used [2] (see the raw data in Table 2.2 and the boxplots in Figure 2.3).

```
> data("acryl", package="SiTuR")
```

Table 2.2: Lung Weight Raw Data in a 13-Week Study on Acrylonitrile

LungWt	dose
0.28	0
0.31	0
0.33	0
0.33	0
0.22	0
...	...
0.19	40
0.20	40
0.30	40
0.21	40
0.26	40

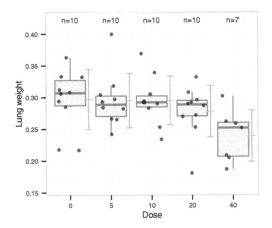

FIGURE 2.3: Boxplots of the lung weight data.

Since the F-test is not significant (p-value of 0.0501), no Dunnett procedure should be used according to the conditional approach mentioned above. But the comparison of the high dose is significant (p-value of the Dunnett procedure of 0.0291). The data are not necessarily normally distributed and a nonparametric approach, i.e., Kruskal—Wallis global test and Steel-type test, reveal a similar behavior ([183]). For endpoints with a directed alternative, the contradiction can even be worse because the quadratic global test is inherently two-sided whereas the Dunnett-type tests can be formulated one-sided. Summarizing, the use of global tests together with Dunnett-type tests cannot be recommended.

2.1.2 Normally distributed continuous endpoints: The Williams procedure

Because the common design in toxicological studies includes dose groups, the assumption of a monotonic increase is appropriate, i.e., a trend alternative should be applied. Again this approach is often used in toxicology: 226 of the 488 citations fall back on the original paper [400] (WebSci January 2014) and recently a 90-day subchronic toxicity study of sodium molybdate dihydrate made use of it [272]. The Williams procedure can be recommended as it is designed for comparisons of several doses versus control (such as Dunnett's procedure), but contains an order restriction. Not only a global trend/no trend decision is possible, but also related simultaneous confidence intervals for pattern-specific information can be derived. The Williams procedure can be formulated as an approximate multiple contrast test with the following contrast matrix in the general unbalanced design [51] (for the sample sizes $n_1, n_2, ..., n_k$):

$$
C = \begin{pmatrix}
C_1 & -1 & 0 & \cdots & 0 & 1 \\
C_2 & -1 & 0 & \cdots & \frac{n_{k-1}}{n_{k-1}+n_k} & \frac{n_k}{n_{k-1}+n_k} \\
\vdots & \vdots & \vdots & \cdots & \vdots & \vdots \\
C_{k-1} & -1 & \frac{n_1}{n_1+...+n_k} & \cdots & \frac{n_{k-1}}{n_1+...+n_k} & \frac{n_k}{n_1+...+n_k}
\end{pmatrix}
\tag{2.2}
$$

Simplified for a balanced design with three dose groups the three contrasts are:

$$
C = \begin{pmatrix}
-1 & 0 & 0 & 1 \\
-1 & 0 & .5 & .5 \\
-1 & .33 & .33 & .33
\end{pmatrix}
\tag{2.3}
$$

The first contrast indicates a strictly global trend by taking into account only the highest dose (with respect to control), the second contrast analyzes the pooled two higher doses, and the third contrast is a plateau of all doses. We can recognize the comparisons-versus-control nature and the robustness against some non-monotonicity by pooling higher doses. The correlation matrix is defined by

$$
\rho_{lm} = \frac{\sum_{i=0}^{k} c_{li}c_{mi}/n_i}{\sqrt{\left(\sum_{i=0}^{k} c_{li}^2/n_i\right)\left(\sum_{i=0}^{k} c_{mi}^2/n_i\right)}} \quad (1 \le l \neq m \le q),
$$

and the approximate $(1-\alpha)100\%$ lower simultaneous confidence limits are

$$
\hat{\delta}_l^{(l)} = \left(\sum_{i=0}^{k} c_{li}\bar{X}_i\right) - t_{k,1-\alpha}(df, \mathbf{R})S\sqrt{\sum_{i=0}^{k} c_{li}^2/n_i} \quad (1 \le l \le q)
$$

with the lower $(1-\alpha)$ quantile $t_{k,1-\alpha}(df, \mathbf{R})$ of the related k-variate t-distribution.

Using the creatine kinase example we expect increasing values with increasing doses. The one-sided lower confidence limits are shown in Figure 2.4 where contrasts are abbreviated C1, ...,C5 according to the contrast matrix in eq. 2.3. All lower limits are larger than the value of H_0 (namely 0) wherein the contrast C1 is the most distant. This suggests a monotonic trend mainly supported by the highest dose 1000 mg/kg. Notice, the object mod1 is the same as for the Dunnett test in the previous section.

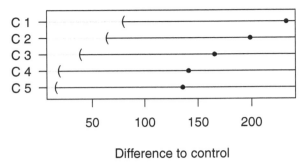

FIGURE 2.4: Williams-type simultaneous confidence limits for serum creatine kinase.

```
> library("multcomp")
> plot(glht(mod1, linfct = mcp(Dose = "Williams"), alternative="greater"),
+       main="", xlab="Difference to control")
```

Please notice, a Williams-type procedure for multiple endpoints is available as well [144]. However, its use in toxicology is limited because of the double union-intersection tests, i.e., the multiplicity adjustment against correlated endpoints and against correlated dose vs. control contrasts is rather conservative even for few endpoints and few dose groups.

2.1.2.1 Dunnett or Williams procedure?

The US NTP recommends Dunnett [102] and Williams [400] test [9], but it does not specify in what situation which of these two should be used. Again the question arises in which situation Dunnett or Williams procedure is appropriate; see also the discussion in [90]. For physiological parameters (type three endpoints in Section 1.2.6) the Dunnett-procedure may be formulated two-sided for a change. The Williams-procedure, however, should be formulated only one-sided for either increasing or decreasing monotonic trends for either endpoint types one and two. The most important advantage of the Williams procedure is the possible claim for a dose-related trend and its (small) power advantage if monotonicity occurs. On the other hand, the Williams procedure cannot claim the difference from dose to control for a single comparison (except for the highest dose) and is not robust for any non-monotonic pattern. Using the concept of claim-wise error rate [301] user-defined Dunnett *and* Williams contrasts were proposed [204] and explained for a balanced design with three doses by its contrast matrix

$$
C = \begin{pmatrix}
Dunnett & -1 & 0 & 0 & 1 \\
Dunnett & -1 & 0 & 1 & 0 \\
Dunnett & -1 & 1 & 0 & 0 \\
Williams & -1 & 0 & 0 & 1 \\
Williams & -1 & 0 & .5 & .5 \\
Williams & -1 & .33 & .33 & .33
\end{pmatrix}
$$

The $(2k - 1)$ contrasts are highly correlated thus the conservatism of its multiple contrast test is not too serious. Claims on either unrestricted or monotonicity-restricted differences to control are possible, which represents a flexible approach for interpretation. For these one-sided comparisons the lower confidence limits are relevant only for endpoints where larger values represent a toxic effect and vice versa. A simple trick in R is used to combine the contrast matrix for Dunnett procedure (cmd) with those of Williams procedure (cmw) into cmdw by the function rbind{}:

```
> library("multcomp")
> ntab <- table(mclinA$Dose)
> cmd  <- contrMat(n=ntab, type="Dunnett")
> cmw  <- contrMat(n=ntab, type="Williams")
> cmdw <- rbind(cmd, cmw)
> plot(glht(model=mod1, mcp(Dose=cmdw), alternative="greater"),
+       main="", xlab="Difference to control", cex.axis=0.65)
```

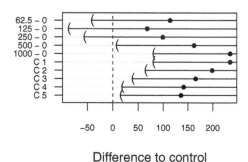

Difference to control

FIGURE 2.5: Simultaneous confidence limits for Dunnett and Williams procedure: creatine kinase example.

In Figure 2.5 we notice first that the contrast C1 (Williams-type) and 1000-0 (Dunnett-type) are the same, namely comparing $\mu_{1000} - 0$. All order restricted contrasts (C1 - C5) are significant, whereas only 1000-0 and 500-0 of the many-to-one (Dunnett-type) comparisons are significant. Clearly most distant from H_0 is the contrast for $\mu_{1000} - 0$. That means the following five claims can be stated: i) an increase against control exists, ii) a trend exists, iii) the trend is mainly supported by the highest dose, i.e the elementary alternative $\mu_C = \mu_{62.5} = ...\mu_{500} < \mu_{1000}$ is likely, iv) all doses above 62.5 contribute to a monotone trend (because their limits are ordered), and v) the no-observed adverse effect level (NOEAL) is 500 (see Section 7 for details).

A further aspect comparing between Williams and Dunnett procedure is the estimation of the lowest observed adverse event level (LOAEL) (see details in Section 7.3).

All order restricted tests based on pooling of groups, such as the Williams test, provide a biased LOAEL estimation [186, 220, 219] and should be avoided. Therefore, the Dunnett procedure can be recommended only for this purpose.

2.1.2.2   A test when downturn effects at high doses seem possible

If the downturn effect at higher doses is serious, e.g., when mutagenic and toxic effects interact in a *in vitro* assay, a downturn protected Williams procedure is available [54]. In a design with k dose groups exactly k peak points ξ are possible, and for each peak point a related Williams contrast can be used. Simplified for a balanced design with $k = 4$ dose groups the contrast matrix is:

$$
C = \begin{pmatrix}
\xi = 4 & -1 & 0 & 0 & 0 & 1 \\
\xi = 4 & -1 & 0 & 0 & .5 & .5 \\
\xi = 4 & -1 & 0 & .33 & .33 & .33 \\
\xi = 4 & -1 & .25 & .25 & .25 & .25 \\
\xi = 3 & -1 & 0 & 0 & 1 & 0 \\
\xi = 3 & -1 & 0 & .5 & .5 & 0 \\
\xi = 3 & -1 & .33 & .33 & .33 & 0 \\
\xi = 2 & -1 & 0 & 1 & 0 & 0 \\
\xi = 2 & -1 & .5 & .5 & 0 & 0 \\
\xi = 1 & -1 & 1 & 0 & 0 & 0
\end{pmatrix}
$$

Because of the high positive correlations between these many contrasts the multiplicity penalty seems to be acceptable. A further view is the downturn-protected combined Dunnett and Williams contrast test [204]. Simplified for a balanced design with $k = 4$ dose groups the contrast matrix is:

$$
C = \begin{pmatrix}
Williams, Dunnett & \xi = 4 & -1 & 0 & 0 & 0 & 1 \\
Williams & \xi = 4 & -1 & 0 & 0 & .5 & .5 \\
Williams & \xi - 4 & -1 & 0 & .33 & .33 & .33 \\
Williams & \xi = 4 & -1 & .25 & 25 & .25 & .25 \\
Williams, Dunnett & \xi = 3 & -1 & 0 & 0 & 1 & 0 \\
Williams & \xi = 3 & -1 & 0 & .5 & .5 & 0 \\
Williams & \xi = 3 & -1 & .33 & .33 & .33 & 0 \\
Williams, Dunnett & \xi = 2 & -1 & 0 & 1 & 0 & 0 \\
Williams & \xi = 2 & -1 & .5 & .5 & 0 & 0 \\
Williams, Dunnett & \xi = 1 & -1 & 1 & 0 & 0 & 0
\end{pmatrix}
$$

From this matrix we can see that several contrasts are the same and hence tested only once. Furthermore, for each possible peak-point, namely $\xi \in (4, 3, 2, 1)$, specific Williams contrasts exist. In addition, the matrix gives an impression of the remarkable correlations. Such a test allows different claims: i) unrestricted Dunnett-type comparisons against control (which could be formulated two-sided also), ii) Williams-type trend comparisons for the complete design, and iii) Williams-type comparisons for all possible peak points (reflecting possible downturn effects at high doses).

As an example, the blood urea nitrogen (BUN) endpoint of the 13-week study with sodium dichromate dihydrate [16] [16] is used, where a non-monotonous dose-response profile is possible; see the boxplots in Figure 2.6.

```
> data("mm", package="SiTuR")
> mm$Dose <-as.factor(mm$Dose)

> mbu <-lm(BUN~Dose, data=mm)
```

The specific contrast matrix is (*abbreviating Du ... Dunnett, Wi ... Williams, U... Umbrella peak-point*):

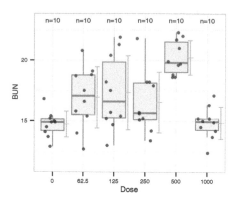

FIGURE 2.6: Boxplots for blood urea nitrogen data.

```
> duwil <- rbind("Du1" = c(-1, 0, 0, 0, 0, 1),
+                "Du2" = c(-1, 0, 0, 0, 1, 0),
+                "Du3" = c(-1, 0,0, 1, 0, 0),
+                "Du4" = c(-1, 0,1, 0, 0, 0),
+                "Du5" = c(-1, 1,0, 0, 0, 0),
+                "Wi2" = c(-1, 0,0, 0, 0.5, 0.5),
+                "Wi3" = c(-1, 0,0, 1/3, 1/3, 1/3),
+                "Wi4" = c(-1, 0,1/4, 1/4, 1/4, 1/4),
+                "Wi5" = c(-1, 1/5,1/5, 1/5, 1/5, 1/5),
+                "U1" = c(-1, 0,0, 0.5, 0.5, 0),
+                "U2" = c(-1, 0, 1/3, 1/3, 1/3, 0),
+                "U3" = c(-1, 1/4, 1/4, 1/4, 1/4,0),
+                "U4" = c(-1, 0, 0.5, 0.5,0, 0),
+                "U5" = c(-1, 1/3, 1/3, 1/3, 0,0),
+                "U6" = c(-1, 0.5, 0.5,0,0, 0))
```

Again, the calculation of the multiplicity-adjusted p-values is simply made by using the function glht with the matrix duwil.

```
> library("multcomp")
> downt <-summary(glht(mbu, linfct=mcp(Dose=duwil), alternative="greater"))
```

Due to limited precision of tiny p-values in Table 2.3, the following classification based on the values of the test statistics t value: i) t_{Du2} is the largest test statistics, i.e., the D_{500} is mostly increased with respect to control, ii) no monotone trend exists because $p_{Du1} = p_{Wi1} > 0.05$, iii) a trend up to D_{500} exists because t_{U1} is the largest test statistics and $p_{U1} < 0.05$ holds true), iv) this trend indicates a plateau containing the doses D_{500}, D_{250}, and v) the LOAEL is D_{125} because $p_{Du4} < 0.05$ but $p_{Du5} > 0.05$. This example demonstrates the possible detailed interpretability of doses against control comparisons.

2.1.3 Normally distributed continuous endpoints: Ratio-to-control procedures

In a repeated toxicity study many endpoints are measured simultaneously and the interpretation of many endpoints with different scales is a challenge. Comparable are si-

Table 2.3: One-Sided Adjusted p-Values for Downturn-Protected Trend Test

Comparison	Test statistics	p-value
Du1	0.1168	0.7964
Du2	5.8164	0.0000
Du3	1.8999	0.1180
Du4	2.7490	0.0197
Du5	2.3351	0.0504
Wi2	3.4255	0.0034
Wi3	3.1978	0.0063
Wi4	3.3463	0.0041
Wi5	3.3352	0.0043
U1	4.4550	0.0001
U2	4.2724	0.0002
U3	4.0478	0.0005
U4	2.6840	0.0230
U5	2.8512	0.0153
U6	2.9353	0.0125

multaneous confidence intervals for ratio-to-control comparisons which can be interpreted as percentage change. Several relevance criteria in toxicology, e.g., the 2-fold rule, are formulated for relative changes as well. The common-used trick, log-transformation of the endpoint and estimation of t-test or Dunnett-intervals (e.g., used by [209]), works only well as long as the endpoint is really log-normal distributed with homogeneous variances. For the common symmetric-distributed endpoints approximate simultaneous confidence intervals are preferable [95]. The related contrast test statistics for the hypotheses $H_{0i} : \frac{\mu_i}{\mu_0} \le \theta$ vs. $H_{1i} : \frac{\mu_i}{\mu_0} > \theta$ is $T_i = \frac{\bar{X}_i - \theta \bar{X}_0}{S\sqrt{\frac{1}{n_i} + \frac{\theta^2}{n_0}}}$

The approximate $(1 - \alpha)100\%$ lower simultaneous confidence limits are:

$$\hat{\theta}_l^{(l)} = \frac{-B_l - \sqrt{B_l^2 - 4A_lC_l}}{2A_l},$$

with

$$A_l = \left(\sum_{i=0}^{k} d_{li} \bar{X}_i \right)^2 - t_{k,1-\alpha}^2 (df, \hat{\mathbf{R}}) S^2 \sum_{i=0}^{k} d_{li}^2 / n_i,$$

$$B_l = -2 \left(\left(\sum_{i=0}^{k} c_{li} \bar{X}_i \right) \left(\sum_{i=0}^{k} d_{li} \bar{X}_i \right) - t_{k,1-\alpha}^2 (df, \hat{\mathbf{R}}) S^2 \sum_{i=0}^{k} c_{li} d_{li} / n_i \right),$$

$$C_l = \left(\sum_{i=0}^{k} c_{li} \bar{X}_i \right)^2 - t_{k,1-\alpha}^2 (df, \hat{\mathbf{R}}) S^2 \sum_{i=0}^{k} c_{li}^2 / n_i$$

where c_{li} and d_{li} are the contrast coefficient in nominator and denominator. Please notice that the elements of the correlation matrix $\hat{\mathbf{R}}$ do not only depend on the contrast coefficients and sample sizes but also on the unknown ratios θ_{i0} where their estimates are plugged-in [95]:

$$\rho_{lm} = \frac{\sum_{i=0}^{k} (c_{li} - \theta_l d_{li}) (c_{mi} - \theta_m d_{mi}) / n_i}{\sqrt{\left(\sum_{i=0}^{k} (c_{li} - \theta_l d_{li})^2 / n_i \right) \left(\sum_{i=0}^{k} (c_{mi} - \theta_m d_{mi})^2 / n_i \right)}} \quad (1 \le l \ne m \le q)$$

A related Williams-type procedure is available as well [184]. Using the R package `mratios` [97] the estimation of simultaneous confidence limits for ratio-to-control comparisons (or multiplicity-adjusted p-values) is straightforward, as demonstrated for the creatine kinase example in a 13-week study [16] (see Figure 2.7).

```
> library("mratios")
> plot(sci.ratio(CreatKinase~Dose, data=mclinA, type="Williams",
+                 alternative="greater"), main="", sub="",
+                 xlab="Ratio-to-control", cex.axis=0.65)
```

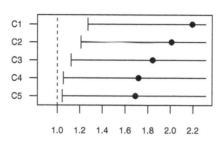

FIGURE 2.7: Simultaneous confidence limits for ratio-to-control Williams-type procedure.

Again, all doses reveal a significant increase against control because they are larger than the value of H_1 (namely 1). For the most significant comparison (highest dose against control) the point estimator is about 2.2-fold and the lower limit about 1.4-fold with respect to control. This multiplicative style is the main difference to the common Dunnett test for differences to control. Here we can interpret a dimensionless increase of at least about 140% creatine kinase increase whereas in the original Dunnett approach an increase of at least 80 units can be interpreted, whatever this means.

2.1.3.1   Procedures when variance heterogeneity occurs

The assumption of a constant coefficient of variation seems to be more plausible in toxicology than the assumption of constant variances with increasing endpoint values or doses. Therefore variance heterogeneity may occur in toxicology naturally. As long as the design is balanced, some degree of heterogeneity is not critical. In this case Dunnett- and Williams-tests are robust. However, when serious variance heterogeneity occurs, and particularly when high variance occurs in groups with small sample sizes, the multiple contrast test with common mean square error estimator is rather conservative [146]. All known standard multiple comparisons procedures (MCP) use pooled variance estimators. For the relevant problem of heteroscedasticity a test statistic with individual variance estimators S_i^2 was proposed [195]. Its generalization for any linear MCP is described [147]:

$$T_l^* = \frac{\sum_{i=1}^k c_{li}\bar{X}_i}{\sqrt{\sum_{i=1}^k c_{li}^2 S_i^2/n_i}} \quad (1 \le l \le q).$$

The exact joint distribution of $(T_1^*, \ldots, T_q^*)$ is not available because the q-variate t-distribution depends on the unknown variances σ_i^2. It can be approximated [147] where each test statistic T_l^* ($1 \leq l \leq q$) is compared with its own distinct quantile coming from a q-variate t-distribution with correlation matrix R (with the elements ρ_{lm}^*) and a Satterthwaite-type calculation of degrees of freedom df_l^* ($1 \leq l \leq q$).

$$df_l^* = \frac{\left(\sum_{i=1}^{k} c_{li}^2 S_i^2 / n_i\right)^2}{\sum_{i=1}^{k} \frac{\left(c_{li}^2 S_i^2 / n_i\right)^2}{n_i - 1}} \quad (1 \leq l \leq q).$$

$$\rho_{lm}^* = \frac{\sum_{i=1}^{k} c_{li} c_{mi} S_i^2 / n_i}{\sqrt{\left(\sum_{i=1}^{k} c_{li}^2 S_i^2 / n_i\right)\left(\sum_{i=1}^{k} c_{mi}^2 S_i^2 / n_i\right)}} \quad (1 \leq l \neq m \leq q).$$

It is important to notice that two modified Dunnett/Williams procedures for heteroscedasticity are available [147, 159]. They can be recommended as THE standard for evaluating approximate normal endpoints analogous to the recommendation of Welch-t-test instead of t-test in the two-sample design as a standard (see above in Section 1.3.1). Since the underlying multivariate t-distribution with an arbitrarily structured correlation matrix is needed, this procedure is numerically available in the R package mratios [121] by means of the function `sci.ratioVH`. The above-mentioned creatine kinase example is analyzed accordingly; see Figure 2.8.

```
> library("mratios")
> plot(sci.ratioVH(CreatKinase~Dose, data=mclinA, type="Williams",
+                  alternative="greater"), main="", sub="",
+                  xlab="Ratio-to-control", cex.axis=0.65)
```

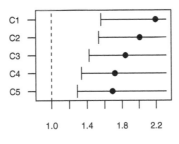

FIGURE 2.8: Simultaneous confidence intervals for ratio-to-control Williams-type procedure allowing heterogeneous variances.

In this example the same conclusion can be drawn assuming homogeneity of variances; see Figure 2.7 and, allowing variance heterogeneity; see Figure 2.8. However, in general the more robust version allowing heterogeneity should be used in routine.

2.1.4   Nonparametric approaches for comparisons versus a negative control

The US National Toxicology Program recommends the evaluation of the majority of variables (such as hematology, clinical chemistry, urinalysis, urine concentrating ability, cardiopulmonary, cell proliferation, tissue concentrations, spermatid, and epididymal spermatozoal data), which have typically skewed distributions, by the nonparametric multiple comparison methods of Shirley (1977) [356] and Dunn (1964) [101]. Hereby, the Shirley procedure assumes an order restriction, whereas the Dunn procedure is the nonparametric analogue of the Dunnett procedure. The nonparametric analysis in one-way layouts has to be distinguished firstly into pairwise-ranking (Wilcoxon rank sums) and joint-ranking approaches (Kruskal–Wallis ranking), whereas both approaches are equivalent only asymptotically. Furthermore, they can be distinguished into tests for the shift alternative and the alternative for relative effects. Since our objective is a nonparametric Behrens–Fisher procedure (Notice, Behrens and Fisher first described the variance heterogeneity problem, whereas Welch published the first solution, still used today), we focus on a joint-ranking approach for relative effects. Their null hypothesis $H_0 : p = \frac{1}{2}$ can be tested for two independent random variables X_1 and X_2 with distributions F_1 and F_2 for the relative treatment effect: $p_{12} = Pr(X_1 < X_2) + \frac{1}{2}Pr(X_1 = X_2) = \int F_1 dF_2$ [62]. Equivalently $l \in (1, ..., q)$ multiple contrasts can be formulated for the pooled samples in a one-way layout: $p_l = \int (\sum |c_{li}| F_i) d(\sum c_{lj} F_j)$, where the contrast matrix is analogous to the parametric case; see for details Section 2.1.1. The single test statistic is: $T_l = \sqrt{N} \frac{\hat{p}_l - 0.5}{\sqrt{\hat{\nu}_l}}$, whereas for the maximum test $T_{max} = max(T_1, ..., T_q)$ the $T_1, ..., T_q$ follows jointly an approximate q-variate normal distribution $z_{q, two-sided, 1-\alpha, R}$ with correlation matrix R. This correlation matrix is estimated from the sample sizes, the particular chosen contrast coefficients (as in the parametric model) and the sample specific variances [225]. Therefore, they commonly do not have a product-moment structure. For small sample size an approximate t-distributed Behrens–Fisher version with a related estimated degree of freedom df^* [62] is highly recommended. Related confidence intervals are available:

$$Pr\left(\hat{p}_l - t_{k,df^*,two-sided,1-\alpha,R}\sqrt{\frac{\nu_l}{N}} \leq p_l \leq \hat{p}_l + t_{k,df^*,two-sided,1-\alpha,R}\sqrt{\frac{\nu_l}{N}} \right) \rightarrow (1-\alpha)$$

whereas a range $[0, 1]$ preventing transformations can be recommended, e.g., the logit transformation. A related R package `nparcomp` [230] is available. For the previous creatine kinase example, let us assume that approximate normal distribution for the error of the endpoint creatine kinase cannot be considered, and thus the nonparametric Dunnett-type intervals should be used instead:

```
> library("nparcomp")
> creatNP <-nparcomp(CreatKinase~Dose, data=mclinA, type="Dunnett",
+                    asy.method = "mult.t",alternative = "greater",
+                    plot.simci =FALSE, info = FALSE,correlation=TRUE)
> CRK <-creatNP$Analysis$Estimator
> names(CRK) <-creatNP$Analysis$Comparison
> CRKlower <-creatNP$Analysis$Lower
> CRKupper <-creatNP$Analysis$Upper
> library("MCPAN")
> plotCII(estimate=CRK, lower=CRKlower, upper=CRKupper,
+         xlab="Relative effect size [0,1]",
+         lines=0.5, lineslty = 3, cex.axis=0.65)
```

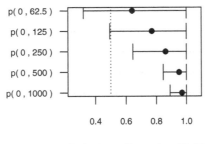

Relative effect size [0,1]

FIGURE 2.9: Simultaneous confidence intervals for relative effect sizes.

Again, by means of the function `nparcomp` and the matrix type `"Dunnett"` the simultaneous confidence limits can be easily estimated. Alternatively multiplicity-adjusted p-values can be estimated. In Figure 2.9 the related lower one-sided limits are depicted. Notice, the value of H_0 is 0.5 and the order of comparisons on the y-axis is reverse to those for the parametric approach (e.g., in Figure 2.8). In contrast, more important is the robustness against non-normality and variance heterogeneity. Furthermore, the confidence intervals for relative effect size allow an individual-based interpretation. For example, the probability of any future single animal in the highest dose (1000) revealing higher value of creatine kinase than any in the control is 78.7%. A related Williams-type trend test- a modification of the Shirley trend test [356] is available as well [228] using the contrast option `"Williams"` in the function `nparcomp` [230]. Because of the pooled groups, an individualized interpretation may be difficult, and therefore the related adjusted p-values are recommended for interpretation. Notice that Shirley's trend test is commonly used in toxicology: it is mentioned in 119 of the 207 citations of the original paper [356] (WebSci January 2014) or recently in a subchronic inhalation toxicity study of fuel oxygenate vapors [78].

2.1.5 Simultaneous comparisons versus a negative control for proportions

The analysis of proportions, as well as the analysis of graded histological findings, belongs to the most important evaluations of a toxicological study because their predictive value is commonly high. Paradoxically, their statistical evaluation can be rarely found in study reports, e.g., hematological endpoints and organ weights were statistically analyzed in a 28-day study for a possible effect of BaSO4 nanoparticles on rats, but not the incidences of inflammatory cell infiltrates in the submucosa of the glandular stomach (Table 9 in [64]). For the analysis of incidences of neoplasms or non-neoplastic lesions, the US NTP [9] recommends an arcsine transformation *"...to bring the data into closer conformance with a normality assumption."* However, the arcsine transformation is not appropriate for small sample sizes [71], particularly for zero cells [327], and therefore alternatives should be used. However, the global rejection of arcsine transformation [388] is a bit excessive. Nevertheless, related transformation approaches are described in the following subsection below. To make matters worse, complex designs and data conditions make the selection of an appropriate procedure for proportions a challenge.

First, two quite different data models should be distinguished: i) the event $(0, 1)$ is measured on the level of the randomized unit (e.g., animal), which results in a 2-by-k table data structure (e.g., for crude tumor incidences), and ii) for each randomized unit a proportion is measured, which binomial data with possible overdispersion exists (e.g., the number of micronucleated erythocytes per scored polychromatic erythrocytes within a single mouse in the *in vivo* micronucleus assay [176]). Unfortunately, most statistical publications focus on the analysis of 2-by-2 or 2-by-k table data, but proportions in toxicology are commonly overdispersed. In the following, small-sample Dunnett/Williams-type one-sided confidence limits for 2-by-k table data are proposed. The specific approaches for overdispersed data are described in Section 2.1.5.4.

Second, mostly asymptotic approaches are used, i.e., defined for large sample sizes. The difference to other asymptotic tests, such as the Wilcoxon test is, that for much higher sample sizes, compliance with the nominal coverage probability is achieved. The rule of thumb is $n_i > 10$ for application of nonparametric tests, but $n_i > 40$ for application of adjusted intervals on proportions [60] where asymptotic methods can be used approximately. But the common sample sizes in toxicological assays is much smaller: about $n_i = 50$ in long-term carcinogenicity assays, $n_i = 20$ in 90 days bioassays and even $n_i = 5$ in *in vivo* mutagenicity assays. These small sample sizes cause two serious problems: the common phenomenon of small power and exceeding or failing of the level α.

Third, (near-to) zero value(s) in the control may cause statistical problems. Ironically, this is exactly the ideal situation for pathological endpoints, such as spontaneous incidences of rare tumors.

Fourth, several effect sizes should be distinguished for proportions: risk difference, risk ratios, and odds ratios. The odds ratio is appropriate for the evaluation of case-control designs, commonly used in epidemiology and genetics. In toxicology however, animals are randomized to the dose group. In contrast, in case-control designs, cases are matched to controls and later the levels of the factor are found experimentally, e.g., the three groups in genetic association studies: homozygote risk allele, heterozygote and homozygote non-risk alleles [177]. Unfortunately, many recent statistical publications deal with case-control designs. Furthermore, the (log) odds ratio is here the natural effect size when using the generalized linear model (GLM) and the logit link (see below). Notice, risk and odds ratio behave similarly only for small p_i and large n_i, which do not necessarily occur in toxicological bioassays. Numerous approaches were worked out to solve the basic dilemma of the obvious GLM approach, namely an unusual effect size, and a liberal behavior for small sample sizes particularly when zeros occur in the control. But so far, no gold standard has been established, i.e., it remains a difficult choice of the less bad variant. A recently developed profile likelihood approach [124] can overcome the difficulties for small sample designs with effect sizes near to 0 or 1 for any link function in the GLM; see the alveolar/bronchiolar tumors example [310] below.

Fifth, for the proportion-generating pathological endpoints one-sided confidence limits (respective tests) are commonly appropriate, i.e., lower limits for the proof of hazard and upper limits for the poof of safety. Because proportions are defined between 0 and 1, one-sided limits are not simply the $(1-\alpha)$ instead of $(1-\alpha/2)$ intervals of the t-test. Specific one-sided approaches are needed; see e.g., [340].

Sixth, exact (permutation) tests derived historically from the analysis of a 2-by-2 table, namely Fisher's exact test is in wide spread use. To overcome the conservativeness of such conditional tests, unconditional tests were established and a related Dunnett-type test is available in the R package `binMto` [221, 349]. Recently an unconditional version of Bartholomew's E_k^2 (see Section 2.2) was made available [81] however without available software.

Seventh, the analysis of multiple binary data can be relevant, such as the number of skeletal and organ malformations; see Section 2.1.5.5.

2.1.5.1   Analysis of 2-by-k table data using the generalized linear model (GLM)

The basics for the generalization of simultaneous inference to the generalized linear model, i.e., for proportions and counts instead of normal distributed endpoints, are the asymptotic concepts for several parametric and semiparametric models, such as generalized linear models, mixed effect models, models for censored data, etc. [189, 55]. The term *asymptotic* implies sufficient large sample sizes, which is commonly violated for proportions in toxicology (see above). In the following, this method is explained for 2-by-k table data using as an example the incidences of tubular epithelia hyaline droplet degeneration (endpoint `tehdd`) in male rats: $0/10, 0/10, 3/10, 8/10$ in [407]; see Table 2.4.

Table 2.4: Incidences of Tubular Epithelia Hyaline Droplet Degeneration: 2-by-4 Table Data

Comparison	Dose	0	D10	D50	D100
Without		10	10	7	2
With		0	0	3	8

First, a generalized linear model should be fitted using the link function `logit`, where the dichotomous endpoint consists of responder (`tehdd`) and non-responder (`no`):

```
> tubuG <- glm(degen ~ Dose, data=tubular, family= binomial(link="logit"))
```

The object `tubuG` is used within the `glht` function:

```
> library("multcomp")
> tubuCI <- glht(tubuG, linfct = mcp(Dose="Dunnett"),alternative="greater")
```

Table 2.5: Summary Statistics of Dunnett-Type Analysis of a 2-by-k Table

Comparison	p-value
D10 - 0	0.625
D50 - 0	0.623
D100 - 0	0.623

The multiplicity-adjusted p-values in Table 2.5 are surprisingly rather large. The reason for this and therefore a serious limitation of this approach can be seen from the estimated huge log-odds ratios and their standard errors caused by the zero cells (and the small sample sizes). Actually, the log-odds ratio in the object `tubuCI` will be re-transformed, but because of the inappropriate estimates, the odds ratios and their lower limits are unsuitable (Table 2.6):

To demonstrate the impact of this zero-cell effect, the analysis is repeated with manipulated data; therefore zeros are replaced by 1. Now, seemingly nice estimators and limits result

Table 2.6: Biased Estimates and Confidence Intervals

Comparison	Odds ratio	Lower confidence limit
D10 - 0	1.00	0.00
D50 - 0	134728292.23	0.00
D100 - 0	1257464060.78	0.00

in Table 2.7. Nevertheless, their coverage probability is vague because of the small sample sizes.

Table 2.7: Add1-Adjusted Estimates and Intervals

Comparison	Odds ratio	Lower confidence limit
D10 - 0	1.00	0.05
D50 - 0	3.86	0.30
D100 - 0	36.00	2.48

Therefore, for proportions in toxicology, organized in 2-by-k tables, the above GLM-approach cannot be recommended. Notice, the use of the GLM-approach for possibly overdispersed data is discussed in Section 2.1.5.4.

2.1.5.1.1 Dunnett-type test using a profile likelihood approach When Wald-type intervals in the GLM are problematic, e.g., in the case of near-to-zero proportions in the control and small sample sizes, likelihood profiles based on signed root likelihood statistics can improve the properties of simultaneous confidence intervals [124]. As an example the crude incidences of hepatocellular carcinoma in the NTP bioassay on methyleugenol (No. TR491) in female mice was selected [314] (see further details in Section 3.6.1).

```
> data("miceF", package="SiTuR")
```

Table 2.8: 2-by-4 Table Data of Hepatocellular Carcinoma

Dose	Without tumor	With tumor
0	50	0
1	26	24
2	21	29
3	12	38

The 2-by-4 table data are in Table 2.8 where the incidence in the control is 0. Particularly for tumor rates with zero tumors in the control a certain specification is needed in which the likelihood is evaluated by means of the argument (`cgrid`).

```
> library("multcomp")
> library("mcprofile")
> library("ggplot2")
```

```
> CM <- contrMat(table(mice29$Group), type="Dunnett")
> mG29 <- glm(t29 ~ Group-1, data = mice29, family = binomial())
> waldci <-fortify(confint(glht(mG29, linfct=mcp(Group="Dunnett"),
+                           alternative = "greater")))
> cgrid <- sapply(1:nrow(CM), function(i) seq(-10, 10, length=100))
> mpCI29 <- mcprofile(mG29, CM, grid=cgrid) ## profile L.
> mcC <- confint(mpCI29, alternative = "greater")$confint
```

Table 2.9: Wald-Type vs. Signed Root Profile Likelihood Confidence Limits

Comparison	Odds Ratio	Lower limit GLM	Lower limit Profile L.
1 - 0	18.5	-1498.8	3.5
2 - 0	18.9	-1498.4	3.9
3 - 0	19.7	-1497.6	4.7

The object `waldci` contains the non-estimable Wald-type intervals (with the incorrect conclusion of no effect at all), whereas the object `mcC` contains the estimates for the modified approach. The estimates for the odds ratio for all three doses with respect to control are rather large, their lower confidence limit reveals strong increasing incidences of hepatocellular carcinoma.

2.1.5.2 Analysis of 2-by-k table data using exact procedures

For 2-by-k table data conditional and unconditional exact Dunnett-type approaches are discussed here; providing adjusted p-values, but no simultaneous confidence intervals. The package `coin` provides conditional inference (so called permutation tests) for continuous, categorical, and censored data for two- and k-sample oneway layouts. As an example the incidences of tubular epithelia hyaline droplet degeneration are used (see Table 2.4).

```
> library("coin")
> library("multcomp")
> duC <- function(data) trafo(data, factor_trafo = function(x)
+ model.matrix(~x - 1) %*% t(contrMat(table(x), "Dunnett")))
> dutub <-independence_test(degen ~ Dose, data = tubular,
+               teststat = "maximum", distribution = "approximate", xtrafo=duC,
+               alternative="less")
> pvalCODU <-pvalue(dutub, method="single-step")
```

A Dunnett-type test is used, where the three multiplicity-adjusted p-values are for the comparison against the low dose 0.812 against medium dose 0.245 and against the high dose 10^{-4}. Notice, the library `coin` provides an exact conditional approach for two-sample tests only; therefore for this k-sample design the approximated distribution with 1000 Monte Carlo replications is used. By the argument `xtrafo` the Dunnett contrasts are invoked.

Unconditional exact tests provide a higher power which is calculated by maximizing the tail probability over the complete domain of the unknown nuisance parameter, i.e., on the observed marginal totals.

```
> library("binMto")
> pKoch <-ec.mto(n=c(10,10,10,10), x=c(0,0,3,8),alternative= "greater")
```

A related Dunnett-type approach is available [221], where in the package `binMto` the p-value for the global maximum test is available using the function `ec.mto` (6.91×10^{-5}).

2.1.5.3 Analysis of 2-by-k table data using adjusted cell estimates

Incidence of macro- and microscopic findings belongs to the second endpoint type, and therefore one-sided lower confidence limits for a possible increase should be considered, whereas the approach should be robust for possible near-to-zero proportions in the control. Simultaneous confidence limits for differences of proportions versus control is a challenge for both small and moderate sample sizes commonly used in toxicology. For one-sided simultaneous limits a simple *adding 0.5 success and 0.5 failure* (denote as ADD-1) approach reveals the best coverage probability for near-zero spontaneous rates [346]. Let Y_i be independent binomial random variables $Y_i \sim Bin(n_i, \pi_i)$, $i = 1, ..., I$, with point estimators $p_i = Y_i/n_i$. Let $C = (c_1, ..., c_I)$ be a vector of appropriate contrast coefficients fulfilling the constraint $\sum_{i=1}^{I} c_i = 0$. Then the $(1 - \alpha)100\%$ approximate lower simultaneous limit is: $\sum_{i=1}^{I} c_{im} \tilde{p}_i - q_{M,R,1-\alpha} \sqrt{\sum_{i=1}^{k} c_{im}^2 \tilde{V}(p_i)}$ with approximated estimators: $\tilde{p}_i = \frac{Y_i + 0.5}{n_i + 1}$ and variance estimators $\tilde{V}(p_i) = \tilde{p}_i (1 - \tilde{p}_i)/(n_i + 1)$ where $q_{M,R,1-\alpha}$ is the equicoordinate $(1 - \alpha)$ quantile of a M-variate normal distribution with correlation matrix R. Again, the correlation matrix depends not only on the contrast coefficient and sample sizes, but also on the variances $\tilde{V}(\tilde{p}_i)$ [52]. Other contrast formulations, such as Williams-type comparisons, behave similarly in this approximate approach [346]; see below. For the three effect sizes: risk difference, risk ratio, and odds ratio approximate Dunnett-type approaches and their simultaneous confidence intervals are available using the package MCPAN. In case of one-sided lower limits the Add1-approach can be recommended for risk differences [346, 22, 313] (using the option `method=ADD1`), risk ratios [120], and odds ratios [234] (using the option `method=Woolf`). Because ratio-to-control inference is considered as well, as an example the manipulated non-zero cell incidences of tubular epithelia hyaline droplet degeneration is used (see Table 2.4).

```
> library("MCPAN")
> degenM <-c(0,0,3,8)
> animals <-c(10,10,10,10)
> dosesN <- c("0", "10", "50", "100")
> degenRD <-binomRDci(n=animals, x=degenM, names=dosesN,
+                     alternative="greater", method="ADD1", type="Dunnett")
> degenRR <-binomRRci(n=animals, x=degenM, names=dosesN,
+                     alternative="greater", type="Dunnett")
> degenOR <-binomORci(n=animals, x=degenM, names=dosesN,
+                     alternative="greater", method="Woolf", type="Dunnett")
```

The three patterns of the lower limits look similar at first glance (Figure 2.10) and they reveal also the same decision, i.e., only the proportion in the 100 mg/kg dose group is significantly increased against control. However, the $H_0 = 0$ for risk difference, but $H_0 = 1$ for risk and odds ratio. Although we see a remarkable 17-fold increase in proportions of the high dose, its lower limit is only 0.92, questioning whether this significant increase is also a biologically relevant increase.

Related Dunnett/Williams-Type confidence limits for mortality-adjusted tumor rates, poly-3 estimates, are described in Section 3.5.

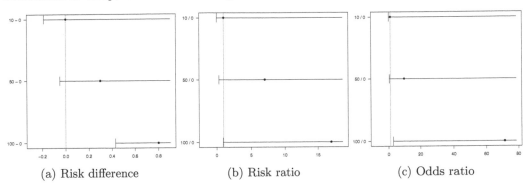

(a) Risk difference   (b) Risk ratio   (c) Odds ratio

FIGURE 2.10: Simultaneous lower confidence limits for adjusted proportions.

2.1.5.4   Analysis of overdispersed proportions

It is important to distinguish designs where i) a proportion is estimated on the treatment level only, e.g., histopathological incidences in long-term studies or tumor rates in carcinogenicity studies and ii) a proportion is estimated on each animal-level, so that a variability between the animals within each treatment group should be taken into account, e.g., the proportions of micronuclei/polychromatic erythrocytes per animal of an *in vivo* micronucleus assay or the proportions of dead fetuses within a litter. Several statistical models can be used to model this between-animal variability, which is referred to as overdispersion in the case of proportions and counts. Here, we analyze example data using i) the generalized linear model with the `quasibinomial(link="logit")` link function, ii) the generalized mixed effect model with a random factor for the between-animal variability and, iii) the simple arcsine square root transformation (arcsine). Particularly for the common small sample sizes used in toxicology, the model choice is still a challenge. As an example we use an aquatic bioassay on aflatoxin (available in the R package **gpk** [371]), where the number of fish with tumors and the total number of fish for four tanks are available; see the raw data in Table 2.10. The between-animal variability is rather specific here as a between-tank variability.

```
> data("fishtoxin", package="gpk")
```

Table 2.10: Raw Data of Aquatic Bioassay on Aflatoxin

Dose	Aflatoxin	Tank1	Tank2	Tank3	Tank4
0.01	with tumor	9	5	2	9
0.01	total count	87	86	89	85
0.02	with tumor	30	41	27	34
0.02	total count	86	86	86	88
0.05	with tumor	54	53	64	55
0.05	total count	89	86	90	88
0.10	with tumor	71	73	65	72
0.10	total count	88	89	88	90
0.25	with tumor	66	75	72	73
0.25	total count	86	82	81	89

However, such a data structure is inappropriate for transformed data in a GLM. Therefore, using the functions `melt, dcast` in the package `reshape2` (see R-details in Appendix A) the data are rearranged into columns for all factors (i.e., conversion from wide to long data format), subject-identifiers, covariates, variables and rows for individuals (animals, but even replicates within an animal), and complete data as possible (see Table 2.11, where `AS` stands for arcsine-transformed tumor rate). Notice, `dose` is a factor, instead of the covariate `Dose`.

```
> library("reshape2")
> fish <- melt(fishtoxin, c("Dose", "Aflatoxin"))
> fishT <- dcast(fish, Dose + variable ~ Aflatoxin)
> colnames(fishT) <-c("Dose", "Tank", "Count", "Tumor")
> fishT$dose <-as.factor(fishT$Dose)
> fishT$AS <-asin(sqrt(fishT$Tumor/fishT$Count))
```

Table 2.11: Structured Aflatoxin Raw Data

Tank	Count	Tumor	dose	AS
Tank1	87	9	0.01	0.33
Tank2	86	5	0.01	0.24
Tank3	89	2	0.01	0.15
Tank4	85	9	0.01	0.33
Tank1	86	30	0.025	0.63
...	...	...	...	...
Tank3	81	72	0.25	1.23
Tank4	89	73	0.25	1.13

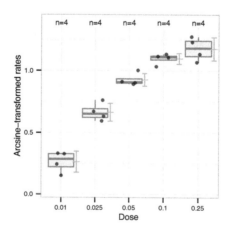

FIGURE 2.11: Boxplots of arcsine transformed data of aflatoxin bioassay.

The boxplots of the arcsine-transformed endpoint (see Figure 2.11) show a serious increasing effect with increasing doses. However, in this example no control data are available, and therefore all-pairwise comparisons (option `"Tukey"`) were used in the following approaches.

Table 2.12: Adjusted Tukey-Type p-Values for Three Approaches Taking Overdispersion into Account

Comparison	Mixed model	GLM	Arcsine
0.025 - 0.01	0	0	0.00013
0.05 - 0.01	0	0	0
0.1 - 0.01	0	0	0
0.25 - 0.01	0	0	0
0.05 - 0.025	9e-04	6e-06	0.000812
0.1 - 0.025	0	0	1e-06
0.25 - 0.025	0	0	1.5e-05
0.1 - 0.05	0.348551	0.136643	0.003935
0.25 - 0.05	0.112431	0.020227	0.007647
0.25 - 0.1	0.975246	0.942691	0.671771

2.1.5.4.1 Generalized mixed effect model An obvious approach is the generalized mixed effect model. The between-tank variability is modeled in the function `glmer` by the random factor `(1tank)|` and the proportion is modeled by `family=binomial(link="logit")`. Care is needed for three items: `dose` must be a factor, the proportion is defined by `cbind(success, failure)` (not by `cbind(success, total number)`). The factor `tank` must have 20 different levels, since there are 5 dose groups and 4 tanks per dose group. In other words, each tank needs to be assigned a unique identifier (here `letters [1:20]` are used, not the inappropriate same levels `tank1`, `tank2`, `tank3`, `tank4` for each treatment).

The related object `fitmMF` is plugged-in to an all-pair comparison procedure ("Tukey") where the related adjusted p-values are calculated (Table 2.12).

```
> library("multcomp")
> library("lme4")
> fishT$tank <-factor(letters[1:20])
> fitmMF <- glmer(cbind(Tumor, Count) ~ dose-1 + (1|tank), data=fishT,
+               family=binomial(link="logit"))
> mMP <-summary(glht(fitmMF, linfct = mcp(dose = "Tukey")))
```

2.1.5.4.2 Generalized linear model with overdispersion The common way to analyze overdispersed proportions is the generalized linear model with the link function `quasibinomial(link="logit")`, allowing the estimation of a dispersion parameter. Using the object containing its estimates (`ovDU`) with the `glht` function provides the estimation of simultaneous confidence limits or adjusted p-values.

```
> library("multcomp")
> ovDu <-glm(cbind(Tumor, Count) ~ dose, data=fishT,
+           family=quasibinomial(link="logit"))
> ovMP <-summary(glht(ovDu, linfct = mcp(dose = "Tukey")))
```

The object `ovMP` contains the adjusted p-value for all-pairs comparisons. Both methods, the generalized mixed effect model in Section 2.1.5.4.1 and the generalized linear model in Section 2.1.5.4.2 reveal similar p-values in this particular example.

2.1.5.4.3 Arcsine square root transformation approaches The US NTP [9] proposed the arcsine transformation for the evaluation of proportions. This is a simple approach

[135] and allows large-sample size tests for both differences and ratios of proportions. Because their confidence intervals are hard to interpret, we focus on multiplicity-adjusted p-values instead. Notice, this transformation is particularly suitable for overdispersed proportions, because for each animal a proportion will be transformed.

```
> library("multcomp")
> fishM <-lm(AS~dose, data=fishT)
> library("sandwich")
> fis <-summary(glht(fishM, linfct=mcp(dose = "Tukey"),vcov=vcovHC))
```

Be careful with these approaches, since their small sample behavior with near-to-zero control proportions is not known (see for example two-sample tests [340]).

2.1.5.5   Analysis of multiple binary data

Multiple binary data occur in toxicology, e.g., multiple tumors in long-term carcinogenicity studies (see Section 3.6.1) or multiple malformation findings in reproductive toxicity studies (see Section 5.3.2). Commonly, these proportions are analyzed independently, each at level α. Some approaches for jointly analyzing multiple binary data exist [87, 24, 265]. However, the related R-code is still missing. Therefore, we focus on a maximum test [218], extended to k-sample layout. Because of the problematic correlation between binary endpoints, such an approach is only slightly more powerful than a simple Bonferroni approach. Moreover, its correlation matrix is difficult to estimate. A simpler solution is to consider endpoint-specific generalized linear models and to derive the correlations between test statistics through asymptotic arguments [307]. Accordingly, the data example used in [218] was re-analyzed by the function mmm in the R-package multcomp (see the documentation).

2.1.6   Trend tests for proportions

2.1.6.1   Cochran–Armitage trend test

Trend tests for proportions are quite commonly used in toxicology, e.g., incidences or poly-3 estimates are mostly tested by the Cochran–Armitage trend test (CA-test). This test is a Wald test for linear regression for proportions and therefore sensitive for near-to-linear shapes of the dose-response relationship. This test is not powerful for either concave or convex shapes, which can be problematic in toxicology. Its data model is a 2-by-k table, i.e., overdispersion for replicated proportion within an experimental unit is ignored. Both an asymptotic and an exact version exist as well as a one-sided and a two-sided version (whereas the restriction to an ordered, even linear, alternative without a directional restriction is hard to imagine). No confidence intervals are available and a challenging problem is the optimal choice of scores, i.e., the values assigned to the dose groups (see Section 2.1.6.2). Furthermore, adjustment against covariates is problematic. Again, we use as example data the 2-by-k table of tubular epithelia hyaline droplet degeneration; see Table 2.4. The package coin provides conditional inference for categorical data for k-sample oneway layouts and will be used in four modifications.

```
> library("coin")
> int1 <-independence_test(degen ~ Dose, data = tubular,
+   teststat = "maximum", distribution = "asymptotic",
+   alternative="less", scores = list(Dose = c(0, 1,  2, 3)))
> pCA <-pvalue(int1)
```

```
> int2 <-independence_test(degen ~ Dose, data = tubular,
+        teststat = "maximum", distribution = "asymptotic",
+   alternative="less", scores = list(Dose = c(0, 0,  0, 1)))
> pcC <-pvalue(int2)
> duD <- function(data) trafo(data, factor_trafo = function(x)
+ model.matrix(~x - 1) %*% t(contrMat(table(x), "Dunnett")))
> dutub <-independence_test(degen ~ Dose-1, data = tubular,
+        teststat = "maximum", distribution = "asymptotic",
+        xtrafo=duC, alternative="less")
> pdu <-pvalue(dutub, method="single-step")
>
> duW <- function(data) trafo(data, factor_trafo = function(x)
+ model.matrix(~x - 1) %*% t(contrMat(table(x), "Williams")))
> witub <-independence_test(degen ~ Dose-1, data = tubular,
+        teststat = "maximum", distribution = "asymptotic",
+        xtrafo=duW, alternative="less")
> pwi <-pvalue(witub, method="single-step")
```

The CA-test assumes a linear trend using the equidistant scores $(0, 1, 2, 3)$ (for the x data (dose levels)). It reveals a p-value of 1.2×10^{-5} (pCA), whereas a single contrast test for comparing the high dose against control reveals a little lower p-value of 1.1×10^{-5} (pcC), not surprising for these $0/10, 0/10, 3/10, 8/10$ pattern. With a value of 1.07×10^{-4} (in object pD) the related p-value of a Dunnett-type approach is larger, paying the multiplicity price, whereas related p-value of the Williams-type approach is with 8.5×10^{-5} (pwi) again smaller because it assumes monotonicity. Because *a priori* the dose-response shape is unknown, neither the linear trend test nor a test with a particular contrast can be recommended for practical use. Therefore, the Williams-type approach can be suggested.

2.1.6.2 Trend test with optimal dose scores

A further modification of the CA-trend test consists of the selection of optimal dose scores using a maximum test over all possible scores, defined by a certain grid [417]. Using the library(coin) this approach can be easily realized [193, 192, 194]. This will be demonstrated for simple 2-by-3 table data (Table 2.13) from a neurotoxicity study in male rats where the number of rats with stained face was investigated ([368] in their Table 4 without low dose). For the vector of dose scores $0, \kappa, 1$, an optimal κ will be identified.

Table 2.13: 2-by-3 Table Data of a Neurotoxicity Study

	Control	D1	D2
Stained face	0	1	13
No effect	12	11	9

```
> library("coin")
> stain <- as.table(matrix(c( 0,  1, 13, 12, 11, 9), byrow = TRUE, nrow = 2,
+                dimnames = list(Tumor = c("Stained face", "No effect"),
+                Dose = c("Control", "D1", "D2"))))
> sta <- t(stain)
```

```
> gZheng <- function(x) {
+    x <- unlist(x)
+    kappa <- seq(from = 0, to = 1, by = 0.05)
+    tr <- sapply(kappa, function(n) c(0, n, 1)[x])
+    colnames(tr) <- paste("kappa", kappa, sep = "_")
+    tr
+ }
> itstain <- independence_test(sta, xtrafo = gZheng, alternative ="greater")
> pstain <-pvalue(itstain, method = "single-step")
> kappagrid <-kappa <- seq(from = 0, to = 1, by = 0.05)
> plot(kappagrid, pstain, ylab="$p$-value",
>        xlab="Grid for parameter kappa", cex.axis=0.65)
```

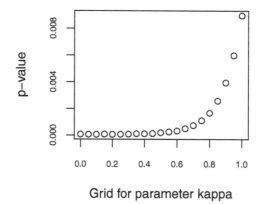

Grid for parameter kappa

FIGURE 2.12: Dependency between the adjusted p-value and the scores parameter.

Figure 2.12 shows the dependency between the adjusted p-value and the scores parameter κ where optimal values are near-to-zero, i.e., most in the alternative is the test for a scores vector of $0, 0, 1$, not surprising when looking at the 2-by-3 table above.

2.1.6.3 Williams-type test using GLM

An alternative is the Williams-type approach in the GLM, similar to the Dunnett-type approach described in Section 2.1.5.1. The three problems: odds ratio as effect size, problems with zero cells, and needed large sample sizes are hidden when using p-values.

2.1.6.4 Williams-type test using adjusted cell estimates

Again, a more robust approach for the incidence data is a Williams-type approach when adding 0.5 success and 0.5 failure (see ADD 1 approach in Section 2.1.5.3). For risk difference, risk ratio, and odds ratio approximate Williams-type approaches are available –either multiplicity-adjusted p-values (for risk difference) and/or simultaneous confidence intervals using the package MCPAN. The ADD-1 approaches are denoted as GNC [120] and Woolf [234]. Again, as an example tubular epithelia hyaline droplet degeneration (2.4) is analyzed.

```
> library("MCPAN")
> ciRD <-binomRDci(degen ~ Dose, success="tehdd", data = tubular,
+           type="Williams",method="ADD1", alternative="greater")
> pvalRD <-binomRDtest(degen ~ Dose, success="tehdd", data = tubular,
+           type="Williams", method="ADD1", alternative="greater")
> ciRR <-binomRRci(degen ~ Dose, success="tehdd", data = tubular,
+           type="Williams", method="GNC", alternative="greater")
> ciOR <-binomORci(degen ~ Dose, success="tehdd", data = tubular,
+           type="Williams", method="Woolf", alternative="greater")
```

Table 2.14: Estimates and Lower Confidence Limits for Williams-Type Approach

	Risk difference	LowerCI RD	Risk ratio	LowerCI RR	Odds ratio	LowerCI OR
C 1	0.80	0.46	17.00	1.41	71.40	3.65
C 2	0.55	0.28	10.91	0.89	26.45	1.60
C 3	0.37	0.16	4.92	0.36	8.88	0.50

The three Williams contrasts reveal rather small p-values in the object pvalRD indicating a strong increasing trend of the tubular epithelia hyaline droplet degeneration incidences. The interpretation of the three Williams-contrasts (C1 against the high dose only, C2 against the pooled high and mid dose, C3 against all pooled doses) for three different effect sizes is specific (see the estimates and the lower confidence limits in Table 2.14) For risk differences all three contrasts are significant, for the risk ratio only the contrast C1 (because the lower confidence limit for C2 is smaller than 1), but for the odds ratio C1 and C2. They all share contrast C1, i.e., a highly significant trend exists dominated by the effect of the high dose group with respect to control, not surprising for these orders of incidences (see Table 2.4). This example highlights the importance of an *a priori* choice of the effect size.

2.1.6.5 Williams-type test using a profile likelihood approach

The recently developed profile likelihood approach [124] is particularly robust for small sample designs. As an example part of the alveolar/bronchiolar tumors example [310] is used (dose groups and tumor indicator).

```
> data("bronch", package="MCPAN")
```

Table 2.15: 2-by-4 Table Data of Alveolar/Bronchiolar Tumors

Dose	Tumors Without	With
0	46	4
1	41	9
2	39	11
3	43	7

The 2-by-4 table (see Table 2.15) shows medium or small sample sizes, a medium spontaneous tumor rate, and a non-monotonic dose-response profile.

```
> library("mcprofile")
> mosaicplot(Tumor ~ group, data = bronch, main="", color=TRUE)
> brGLM <-glm(Tumor ~ group-1, data = bronch, family=binomial())
> library("multcomp")
> CMW <- contrMat(table(bronch$group), type="UmbrellaWilliams")
> brmp <- mcprofile(brGLM, CMW)
> brci <- confint(brmp)
> plot(brci)
```

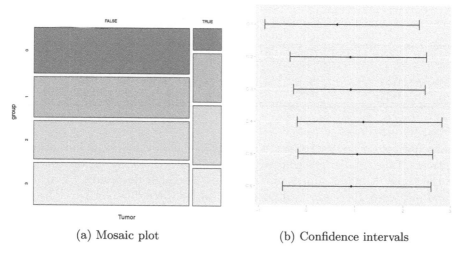

(a) Mosaic plot   (b) Confidence intervals

FIGURE 2.13: Alveolar/bronchiolar tumors example.

Figure 2.13 contains in the left panel the mosaic plot of the proportions and in the right plot the simultaneous confidence intervals for a trend test protected against a downturn effect at higher doses using the profile likelihood approach. The contrast matrix for this downturn protected Williams-type approach is given in Table 2.16:

Table 2.16: Contrasts for Downturn Protected Williams-Type Test

0	1	2	3
-1.00	0.00	0.00	1.00
-1.00	0.00	0.50	0.50
-1.00	0.33	0.33	0.33
-1.00	0.00	1.00	0.00
-1.00	0.50	0.50	0.00
-1.00	1.00	0.00	0.00

2.1.6.6 Trend tests for proportions with possible overdispersion

Overdispersed proportions occur usually in *in vivo* mutagenicity and reproductive assays; for details see Section 4.5. For demonstration purposes two related examples are used, first the proportion of micronuclei/polychromatic erythrocytes per animal of an *in vivo* micronucleus assay with 5-(4-Nitroglycerin)-2,4-pentadien-1-al (NPPD) on the peripheral blood of B6C3F1 mice [7], (see the raw data in Table 4.8) and the number of dead fetuses per number of litter within a female rat (see the raw data in Table 5.3)

```
> data("np", package="SiTuR")
```

```
> library("multcomp")
> np$Risk <-np$PCE-np$MN
> ovWil <-glm(cbind(MN, Risk) ~ Dose, data=np,
+           family=quasibinomial(link="logit"))
> ovCI <- glht(ovWil, linfct = mcp(Dose ="Williams"),alternative="greater")
```

Table 2.17: Williams-Type Analysis of Proportion of Micronuclei per Erythrocytes Taking Overdispersion into Account

Contrasts	Odds ratio	Lower confidence limit
C 1	3.65	2.64
C 2	2.48	1.81
C 3	1.99	1.46
C 4	1.68	1.23
C 5	1.61	1.19

The odds ratios and their lower confidence limits reveal a strong dose-dependent increase in proportion of micronuclei per erythrocytes (see Table 2.17) whereas contrast C1 with the largest confidence limit stands for the likely dose-response pattern, namely caused by the high dose.

The second example (`data(lirat)`) focuses on the number of dead fetuses per number of litter within each female rat whereas unbalanced litter size occurs naturally.

Care is needed when using a generalized linear model with a `quasibinomial(link="logit")` link function because in the data $R = N$ cases exists, i.e., the proportion is on the parameter space. Therefore, the *p*-value in the object `pValuesWIL` may be biased.

```
> library("multcomp")
> ovmp1 <- glm(cbind(R, N-R) ~ treatment-1, data=lirat,
+              family=quasibinomial(link="logit"))
> ovliW <- glht(ovmp1, linfct = mcp(treatment = "Williams"),
+              alternative="less")
> ovliW$df <- df.residual(ovmp1)
> pValuesWIL <-summary(ovliW)
```

2.1.7 Multinomial endpoints: Evaluation of differential blood count

The multinomial distribution is a generalization of the binomial distribution to k categories of events (instead of just two). In toxicology, differential blood count or among others the distribution of mono-, bi-, tri-, and tetra-nucleated cells in the *in vitro* micronucleus assay (see Section 4.13 for details) follow a multinomial distribution. The common independent analysis of each category ignores the specific dependencies between the categories. Multinomial models can be fitted with the add-on package VGAM (vector generalized linear and additive models) [412] which focus on global inference. Simultaneous inference between the dose groups and between the categories can be formulated for specific log odds ratios and its confidence limits using the package mmcp [127, 360]. The approach is conservative because it adjusts against treatment and category comparisons simultaneously. As an example the differential blood counts in a sub-chronic toxicity study on rats is used; see the raw data in Table 2.18 (notice, the original data are presented for 100 total counts). As in the categories basophile granulozytes baso and band neutrophils granulocytes stab only the value 0 occurs they were not considered.

```
> data("dif", package="SiTuR")
```

Table 2.18: Differential Blood Count in Rats

sex	animal	Group	Eos	Baso	Stab	Segm	Mono	Lymph
Males	1101	control	2	0	0	51	2	145
Males	1102	control	3	0	0	28	2	167
Males	1103	control	4	0	0	32	5	159
Males	1104	control	3	0	0	32	6	159
Males	1105	control	8	0	0	30	3	159
Males	1106	control	1	0	0	52	3	144
Males	1107	control	4	0	0	29	3	164
Males	1108	control	4	0	0	23	0	173
Males	1109	control	4	0	0	33	7	156
Males	1110	control	1	0	0	30	1	168
...	...	...	...	...	...	...	...	...
Females	2401	high dose	2	0	0	30	3	165
Females	2402	high dose	1	0	0	22	4	173
Females	2403	high dose	1	0	0	47	1	151
Females	2404	high dose	1	0	0	23	0	176
Females	2405	high dose	2	0	0	19	2	177
Females	2406	high dose	4	0	0	44	6	146
Females	2407	high dose	5	0	0	23	8	164
Females	2408	high dose	4	0	0	14	3	179
Females	2409	high dose	1	0	0	35	4	160
Females	2410	high dose	0	0	0	42	6	152

```
> library("mmcp")
> dbb <- as.matrix(cbind(diff[,c(4,7:9)]))
> colnames(dbb) <- c("Eos","Segm", "Mono", "Lymph")
> multmcp <- multinomMCP(dbb, diff[,3],
+             groups = "Dunnett", endp = "Tukey", char.length=10)
> ci <- confint(multmcp)
> par(cex.axis=0.6)
> par(mar=c(3,8,1,1))
> plot(ci)
```

Figure 2.14 shows the multiple odds ratios: Dunnett-type dose vs. control comparisons, and between each category comparisons $\frac{Pr(Seg)}{Pr(Eos)}, ..., \frac{Pr(Lymph)}{Pr(Mono)}$ where simultaneous confidence intervals are estimated taking the correlations between both treatments and categories into account. In this example almost all confidence intervals contain the value of $H_0 = 1$, but segm shows a significant increase with respect to lymph for the high dose (with respect to control). Notice, this approach allows a k-by-q table data structure, i.e., no overdispersion with non-

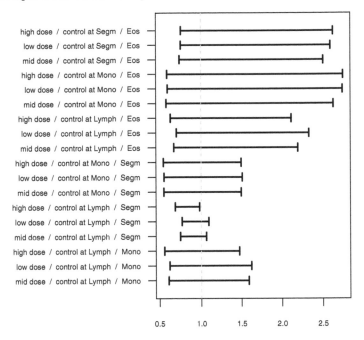

FIGURE 2.14: Simultaneous confidence limits for multiple odds ratios.

zero elements. The differential blood count example and the *in vitro* micronucleus example differ in the definition of between categories comparison. In the first no hierarchy between the categories exists and therefore all-pairs comparisons (Tukey-type) odds ratios are chosen. But in the second the comparisons of bi-, tri-, and tetra-nucleated cells with respect to mono-nucleated cells is of interest and therefore Dunnett-type odds ratios are defined.

2.1.8 Analysis of graded histopathological findings

The evaluation of histopathological findings, particularly those with severity grading, may be highly relevant. However, in some publications these findings are reported without any statistical evaluation, e.g., the acute inflammation in lungs/bronchials [414] or inappropriate methods were used, e.g., the graded findings of basal cell hyperplasia in nonglandular mucosa were analyzed by the Cochran–Armitage test [362]. To explain the specific problems with graded histopathological findings as an example the findings of basophilic tubules in the kidneys of male rats (Table 6 in [407] of a 28-day oral dose toxicity study of nonylphenol is used.

Table 2.19: Graded Histopathological Findings for Basophilic Tubules

Comparison	Dose control	10mgkg	50mgkg	250mgkg
0	10	8	9	0
1	0	2	1	6
2	0	0	0	2
3	0	0	0	2

The raw data are reported in Table 2.19, where the values $0, 1, 2, 3$ represent the degree of severity.

Already from this example six specific conditions for such ordered categorical data can be concluded: i) an effect size reflecting increasing severity with increasing dose is not obvious, ii) the sample size is commonly rather small for such discrete data ($n_i = 10$ rats per group), iii) only one-sided tests or confidence limits are relevant since only increasing severities are of toxicological interest, iv) zero or near-to-zero severity in the control is common for such a pathological endpoint type, v) a few categories are considered, because three to four severity grades can be diagnosed reproducible only, and vi) an increase in variance with dose and/or severity is likely. Therefore, a related statistical approach should be appropriate for these conditions. Several models can be used for ordered categorical data with few categories. Five selected approaches are discussed here: i) data transformation approach (see Section 2.1.9 for details), ii) the generalized linear model assuming a Poisson distribution, whereas extra-Poisson variability between the animals should be considered, iii) a nonparametric Williams-type test for relative effect sizes (see Section 2.1.4 for details), iv) cumulative logit link model, and v) a collapsing categories c-by-k table trend test [133].

(i) Overdispersed near-to-zero counts can be easily transformed into an approximate normal variable using the Freeman–Tukey (FT) root transformation [118, 135] $x_{ij}^{transformed} = \sqrt{x_{ij}} + \sqrt{x_{ij}+1}$ which was used in toxicology for MN counts [179] or number of foci in the cell transformation assay [280]. This transformed variable can be analyzed by Dunnett/Williams test, where adjusted p-values can be recommended, since confidence intervals are hard to interpret in such a transformed scale. The advantage of this simple approach can be demonstrated by the basophilic tubules example because on the control only zero severities occur.

```
> library("multcomp")
> woo$FT <-sqrt(woo$finding)+ sqrt(woo$finding+1)
> library("multcomp")
> modFT <-lm(FT~Dose, data=woo)
> pvalFT <-summary(glht(modFT, linfct=mcp(Dose="Dunnett"),
+                        alternative="greater"))$test$pvalue
```

The p-values for control against dose comparisons are for low dose 0.202, medium dose 0.464, and high dose 10^{-4}, i.e., in the high-dose group significantly higher severities occur compared with the control.

(ii) To demonstrate the use of a generalized linear model, a different data example was selected, where not only zero values in the control occur. For hyaline droplets findings in male rats treated with hexachloro-butadiene [364] four severity scores (1...no abnormality detected; 2... minimal, occasional small hyaline droplets in occasional tubules; 3... mild, scattered small hyaline droplets, 4... moderate, high number of variable sized droplets) were used; see the raw data in Table 2.20.

```
> data("hyalin", package="SiTuR")
```

The mosaic plot in Figure 2.15 shows the specific design using 7 doses and a control and the shift from smaller severities in the control and low dose to higher ones in the higher doses. Because of this somewhat specific design a specific contrast matrix was used for both comparisons against control and Williams-type comparisons for each possible peakpoint; see the related complex contrast matrix in Table 2.21.

Table 2.20: Severity Scores of Hyaline Droplet Degeneration

dose	droplets
0	1
0	1
0	1
0	1
0	2
0	2
5	1
5	1
5	2
5	2
. . .	. . .
45	3
45	4
45	4
45	4
90	3
90	3
90	3
90	4
90	4
90	4

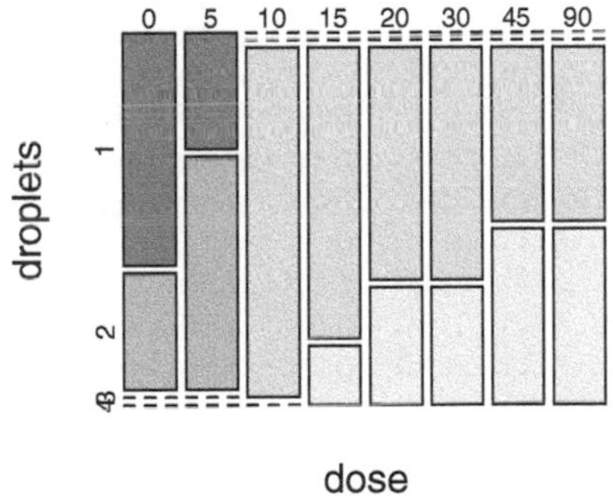

FIGURE 2.15: Mosaic plot of severity scores of hyaline droplets.

```
> exP <-glm(droplets~dose, data=hyalin, family=quasipoisson(link = "log"))
> library("multcomp")
> ntab <- table(hyalin$dose)  # sample sizes needed for unbalanced designs
> cmd <- contrMat(n=ntab, type="Dunnett")
> cmuw <- contrMat(n=ntab, type="UmbrellaWilliams")
> cmduw <- rbind(cmd, cmuw) # combine both matrices
> duw <-summary(glht(exP, linfct=mcp(dose=cmduw),alternative="greater"))
```

In the object duw it can be seen that almost all contrasts are highly significant. Most clearly in the alternative is the contrast C4, reflecting a trend with a plateau including the doses 20, 30, 45, 90.

(iii) The relative effect size approach (see Section 2.1.4) seems to be appropriate for such ordered categorical data [331] as it summarizes the probability that an outcome from a treated distribution exceeds an outcome from the control distribution. It is adjusted for

Table 2.21: Complex Contrast Matrix for Hyaline Droplets Example

	0	5	10	15	20	30	45	90
5 - 0	-1.00	1.00	0.00	0.00	0.00	0.00	0.00	0.00
10 - 0	-1.00	0.00	1.00	0.00	0.00	0.00	0.00	0.00
15 - 0	-1.00	0.00	0.00	1.00	0.00	0.00	0.00	0.00
20 - 0	-1.00	0.00	0.00	0.00	1.00	0.00	0.00	0.00
30 - 0	-1.00	0.00	0.00	0.00	0.00	1.00	0.00	0.00
45 - 0	-1.00	0.00	0.00	0.00	0.00	0.00	1.00	0.00
90 - 0	-1.00	0.00	0.00	0.00	0.00	0.00	0.00	1.00
C 1	-1.00	0.00	0.00	0.00	0.00	0.00	0.00	1.00
C 2	-1.00	0.00	0.00	0.00	0.00	0.00	0.50	0.50
C 3	-1.00	0.00	0.00	0.00	0.00	0.33	0.33	0.33
C 4	-1.00	0.00	0.00	0.00	0.25	0.25	0.25	0.25
C 5	-1.00	0.00	0.00	0.20	0.20	0.20	0.20	0.20
C 6	-1.00	0.00	0.17	0.17	0.17	0.17	0.17	0.17
C 7	-1.00	0.14	0.14	0.14	0.14	0.14	0.14	0.14
C 8	-1.00	0.00	0.00	0.00	0.00	0.00	1.00	0.00
C 9	-1.00	0.00	0.00	0.00	0.00	0.50	0.50	0.00
C 10	-1.00	0.00	0.00	0.00	0.33	0.33	0.33	0.00
C 11	-1.00	0.00	0.00	0.25	0.25	0.25	0.25	0.00
C 12	-1.00	0.00	0.20	0.20	0.20	0.20	0.20	0.00
C 13	-1.00	0.17	0.17	0.17	0.17	0.17	0.17	0.00
C 14	-1.00	0.00	0.00	0.00	0.00	1.00	0.00	0.00
C 15	-1.00	0.00	0.00	0.00	0.50	0.50	0.00	0.00
C 16	-1.00	0.00	0.00	0.33	0.33	0.33	0.00	0.00
C 17	-1.00	0.00	0.25	0.25	0.25	0.25	0.00	0.00
C 18	-1.00	0.20	0.20	0.20	0.20	0.20	0.00	0.00
C 19	-1.00	0.00	0.00	0.00	1.00	0.00	0.00	0.00
C 20	-1.00	0.00	0.00	0.50	0.50	0.00	0.00	0.00
C 21	-1.00	0.00	0.33	0.33	0.33	0.00	0.00	0.00
C 22	-1.00	0.25	0.25	0.25	0.25	0.00	0.00	0.00
C 23	-1.00	0.00	0.00	1.00	0.00	0.00	0.00	0.00
C 24	-1.00	0.00	0.50	0.50	0.00	0.00	0.00	0.00
C 25	-1.00	0.33	0.33	0.33	0.00	0.00	0.00	0.00
C 26	-1.00	0.00	1.00	0.00	0.00	0.00	0.00	0.00
C 27	-1.00	0.50	0.50	0.00	0.00	0.00	0.00	0.00
C 28	-1.00	1.00	0.00	0.00	0.00	0.00	0.00	0.00

ties and allows heterogeneous variance [229]. As a third example for severity findings the non-neoplastic lesions in the p-cresidine carcinogenicity study [201] on each 30 male mice is used. Here, the severity findings of hyperplasia in the parotid gland (salivary glands) is used (where the single finding minimal was categorized as none finding); see the mosaic plot in Figure 2.16.

```
> data("parotid", package="SiTuR")
> paro <-parotid[, 4:5]

> library("nparcomp")
> gradNP <-nparcomp(Score ~Group, data=paro, asy.method = "mult.t",
+ type = "Dunnett", alternative ="greater", plot.simci = FALSE, info=FALSE)
>
> grp <-gradNP$Analysis$Estimator
> names(grp) <-gradNP$Analysis$Comparison
> grplower <-gradNP$Analysis$Lower
> grpupper <-gradNP$Analysis$Upper
```

```
> library("MCPAN")
> plotCII(estimate=grp, lower=grplower, upper=grpupper,
+          xlab="Relative effect size [0,1]",
+          lines=0.5, lineslty=3)
```

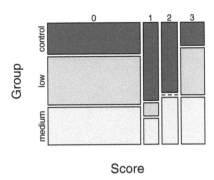

FIGURE 2.16: Mosaic plot for hyperplasia in parotid gland.

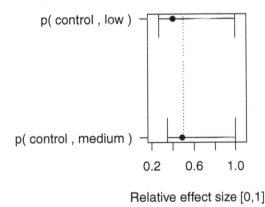

FIGURE 2.17: Nonparametric simultaneous confidence intervals for graded hyperplasia findings.

The lower Dunnett-type confidence limits are presented in Figure 2.17 where the $H_0 = 0.5$ is included in both intervals, i.e., no increase in severity for any dose group can be revealed.

(iv) Cumulative link models
It can be assumed that an ordinal endpoint Z_{ij} falls into $j = 1, \ldots, J$ categories in each of i groups and follows a multinomial distribution with the parameters π_{ij}. Cumulative probabilities $Pr(Z_i \leq j) = \pi_{i1} + \ldots + \pi_{ij}$ can be defined in accord with cumulative logits: $\text{logit}(Pr(Z_i \leq j)) = \log \frac{Pr(Z_i \leq j)}{1 - Pr(Z_i \leq j)}$ can be used within a regression model framework independently for each j by means of the package `ordinal` [77].

As an example liver basophilia severity scores data used in [133] is selected. The raw data are given in Table 2.22.

```
> data("green", package="SiTuR")
> green$dose <-as.factor(green$Dose)
> green$severity <-as.factor(green$Severity)
> green$sever <-as.ordered(green$severity)
> greenTab <-table(green$Dose, green$Severity, dnn=c("Dose", "Severity"))
```

Table 2.22: *c*-by-*k* Table Data of Liver Basophilia Severity Scores

Dose	Severity 1	2	3
1	9	4	1
2	4	8	0
3	7	6	0
4	3	10	1
5	6	4	4

By means of the function `clm` the parameter of a cumulative link model can be fitted whereas the endpoint `sever` is defined as ordered categorical. (The effect size are cumulative log-odds ratios and the parameter estimates are differences to control (abbreviated with 1)). Therefore, Wald-type confidence intervals can be estimated in case Bonferroni adjustments for a Dunnett-type approach were used (level $1 - 0.05/2$ because of 4 comparisons, that are one-sided instead of two-sided); see the lower limits in Table 2.23.

```
> library("ordinal")
> GreenCLM <- clm(sever ~ dose, data=green)
> propCI <-exp(confint(GreenCLM, level=1-0.05/2)) # Bonferroni odds ratio CI
```

Table 2.23: Lower Confidence Limits of Cumulative Link Model in Odds Ratio Scale

	Lower confidence limit
D2 vs. Control	0.47
D3 vs. Control	0.23
D4 vs. Control	0.84
D5 vs. Control	0.66

All simultaneous lower limits are less than one, i.e., no increasing severities from category $1 \Rightarrow 2$ and $2 \Rightarrow 3$ occur in the comparison of any dose with respect to control.

2.1.8.1 Ordered categorical data trend test

(v) Recently, graded histopathological findings were analyzed by a CA-trend test using collapsing categories [133]. The idea is to transform the *c*-by-*k* table data into multiple 2-by-*k* table data in such a way that a trend test reveals the smallest *p*-value. This can be easily explained by the liver basophilia severity scores data used in [133]. The original data with $c = 3$ categories and $k = 5$ dose groups are given in Table 2.22.

Collapsing the scores 1 and 2 into the object S12, as seen in Table 2.24, reveals the smallest

Table 2.24: Collapsed 2-by-k Table Data of Liver Basophilia Severity Scores

Dose	Severity	1	2
1		13	1
2		12	0
3		13	0
4		13	1
5		10	4

p-value for the CA-trend test in [133].

```
> library("coin")
> Gr1 <- independence_test(S12 ~ dose, data = green,
+           scores = list(dose = c(1, 0, 0, 0, -1)), alter = "less")
> pGreen <-pvalue(Gr1, method = "single-step")
```

With these collapsed data and a single contrast test for a convex shape a rather small p-value 0.024 can be achieved applying the permutation test approach. However, statistically it is not a good idea to select data dependent both on a certain collapsing version and on a particular contrast. A solution is to use a Max(Max)-test over both possible collapsing between scores 1 and 2 and 3 and Williams-type comparisons for some shapes of the dose-response relationship (as analogously used in genetic association studies [177]).

```
> gZheng <- function(x) {
+       x <- unlist(x)
+       eta <- seq(from = 0, to = 1, by = 0.1)
+       tr <- sapply(eta, function(n) c(0, n, 1)[x])
+       colnames(tr) <- paste("eta", eta, sep = "_")
+       tr
+ }
>
> w5 <- c(1, 0,0,0,-1)
> w4 <- c(1, 0,0,-1/2,-1/2)
> w3 <- c(1, 0,-1/3,-1/3,-1/3)
> w2 <- c(1, -1/4,-1/4,-1/4,-1/4)
>
> # xtrafo function for independence_test()
> gw <- function(x){
+     x <- unlist(x)
+     cbind(wi5=w5[x], wi4=w4[x], wi3=w3[x], wi2=w2[x])
+ }
>
> itW <- independence_test(severity ~ dose, data = green,
+         ytrafo = function(data) trafo(data, factor_trafo = gZheng),
+         xtrafo = gw, alter = "less")
>
> pvalsMM <-pvalue(itW, method = "single-step")
> MM <-min(pvalsMM)
```

Not surprisingly, the minimum p-value of these many p-values (in object **pvalsMM**) is 0.0798 not significant, as this approach adjusts for 2 collapsings with 4 dose contrasts.

Summarizing, it is difficult to recommend a specific approach. No comparison study exists up to now for data structures typically for graded findings in toxicology. All proposed approaches above suffer from the really unknown behavior for small sample size designs, when only few categories were diagnosed, particularly when zero or near-to-zero findings are in the control. Further work is needed.

2.1.9   Comparisons versus a negative control for transformed endpoints

Data transformation in order to achieve normal distribution and/or homogeneous variances is rather popular: either log-transformed responses and/or log-transformed doses are considered as a *natural* approach in biomedical research. Here, some remarks about data transformations are summarized: First, only for selected transformations a related re-transformation exists, which allows the interpretation in the original effect size. For example, assuming log-normal distribution, re-transformed $(1 - 2\alpha)$ t-test intervals on the log-transformed AUC-endpoints are used to claim bioequivalence for interval inclusion into $[0.8, 1.25]$ [40]. However, care is needed when using log-transformation for any skewed distributed data with possible variance heterogeneity.

Second, a popular alternative to the *a priori* assumption of a particular distribution and homogeneous variances (see Section 2.1.5) is the transformation of the endpoints toward approximately normally distributed variables, such as arcsine transformation (e.g., recommended for the analysis of incidences of non-neoplastic lesions [9]); see for details Section 2.1.5.4.3. Furthermore, overdispersed counts with zero or near-to-zero counts in the control can be transformed into approximate normal variable using the Freeman–Tukey root transformation [118, 135] $x_{ij}^{transformed} = \sqrt{X_{ij}} + \sqrt{X_{ij} + 1}$; see details in Section 2.1.8. Also commonly used is the rank-transformation [79], which was recently used in toxicology [320]). Again, it is a rather simple approach. However, we recommend the nonparametric Dunnett–Williams-type procedure described in Section 2.1.4 instead of rank transformation.

Third, the Box–Cox transformation system can be used [325], a special case of a decision tree approach. In the Box–Cox system $f(y) = \frac{(y+c)^\lambda - 1}{\lambda}$ (where c guarantees positive values) the parameter λ can take any value $[-5, 5]$. It includes $\lambda = 0$ for log-normal transformation, $\lambda = -1$ for reciprocal transformation, $\lambda = -0.5$ for inverse root transformation, $\lambda = -2$ for inverse power transformation, $\lambda = 0.5$ for square root transformation, $\lambda = 2$ for power transformation, and finally $\lambda = 1$ for untransformed data. The problem is to estimate the parameter λ for small sample sizes. As an example for a Box–Cox transformation, the cholesterol endpoint from the 13-week study with sodium dichromate dihydrate to F344 rats [16] is used. Skewness and variance heterogeneity can be seen in the boxplots in Figure 2.18.

```
> data("clin", package="SiTuR")
> clin$dose <-as.factor(clin$Dose)
```

By means of the R package MASS an appropriate λ is estimated for this linear model. Notice, several approaches and related software for λ-estimation are available, but mostly focused on a single variable without any substructure. The function boxcox in the package MASS allows the estimation for a linear model:

```
> library("MASS")
> CholMod <-lm(Cholesterol~dose, data=clin)
> CholLam <-boxcox(CholMod, lambda = seq(-2, 2, length = 100))
> optLam <-CholLam$x[which.max(CholLam$y)]
```

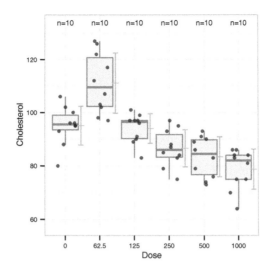

FIGURE 2.18: Boxplots of cholesterol data.

The $\lambda = 0.34$-transformed endpoint is used for a Dunnett-type approach, whereas only adjusted p-values can be used for interpretation (a re-transformation of difference estimates and confidence limits is not possible).

```
> library("hdrcde")
> clin$CholBC <-BoxCox(clin$Cholesterol, lambda =0.3434)
> modCholBC <-lm(CholBC~dose, data=clin)
> library("multcomp")
> CholglhtBC <-summary(glht(modCholBC, linfct=mcp(dose="Dunnett")))
```

The related multiplicity-adjusted p-values for two-sided Dunnett-type tests are represented in Table 2.25.

The adjusted p-values of this Box–Cox transformations in the objects `CholglhtBC` do not differ substantially from related p-values from the nonparametric tests (in the object `pvalCholNP`).

```
> library("nparcomp")
> pvalCholNP <-nparcomp(Cholesterol~dose, data=clin, type="Dunnett",
+            asy.method = "mult.t", plot.simci =FALSE, info = FALSE,
+            correlation=FALSE)$Analysis$p.Value
```

Table 2.25: Box–Cox Transformed and Nonparametric Dunnett-Type Tests on Cholesterol Data

Comparison	p-value Box-Cox	p-value nonpara.
62.5 - 0	0.00054	0.00016
125 - 0	0.99863	1.00000
250 - 0	0.07291	0.04688
500 - 0	0.00579	0.00129
1000 - 0	0.00005	0.00008

All these methods have in common that they are very simple, but that their choice is arbitrary or data-dependent uncertain for designs with small sample sizes as well as hard to interpret [168], and the effect size is no longer in the foreground of interest. It can be helpful, but care is needed.

2.1.10   Testing mixed responder/non-responder data

From the assumption of a tolerance distribution in toxicology [281], a mixture distribution of responder and non-responder subjects also for continuous variables could follow. Two situations should be distinguished: i) small sample designs where even a bi-modal distribution cannot be estimated, but rank-transformation tests for Lehman-alternative can be used, and ii) large sample sizes (at least in the sub-units, such as scored cells) where a mixture distribution can be estimated and the inference focuses only on the responder. A particular simple rank transformation $z_{ij} = (R_{ij}/(N - 1))^3$ can be used [80] (whereas R_{ij} is the rank of observation y_{ij} in the joint sample of i groups and j replicates). The classical Shirley reaction time data are used [356] as example data.

```
> data("reaction", package="nparcomp")
```

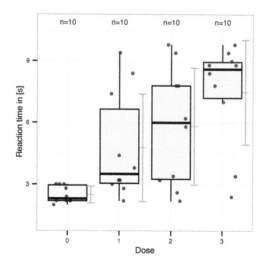

FIGURE 2.19: Boxplots of Shirley's reaction time data.

From the boxplots in Figure 2.19, one could imagine a mixing distribution in the dose groups. To demonstrate the approach, we select a subset of control and the low dose only. The rank transformation followed by the Welch-t-test compared to the Welch-t-test on the original data are compared.

```
> library("nparcomp")
> reaction$Dose <-as.factor(reaction$Group)
> react <-droplevels(reaction[reaction$Dose %in% c(0,1), ])
> react$CSS <-(rank(react$Time)/(length(react$Time)+1))^3
> pCSS <-t.test(CSS~Dose, data=react)$p.value
```

```
> pN <-t.test(Time~Dose, data=react)$p.value
```

The fact that the one p-value of the rank transformation test (0.004) is an order of magnitude smaller than that for the original data (0.022), may be regarded as an indication of a mixing distribution. In any case, this rank-transform test is more sensitive in this example, i.e., the assumption of an unimodal distribution is not always appropriate in toxicology, although used throughout.

2.1.11 Testing non-inferiority: The evaluation of recovery period data

To demonstrate the reversibility of pharmacologically related effects is an important and somewhat undervaluated issue which is of particular interest in sub-chronic studies. Commonly, 50% or less of the animals are observed in a recovery period after substance administration. For non-destructive measured parameters, such as body weight, data both after treatment period and after the recovery period from the same animal are available, i.e., a paired design exists. The claim of recovery can be translated into the proof of equivalence, i.e., a two-sided hypothesis is considered (see Section 2.5.2).

Recovery needs only to be proved for such dose groups, which showed a significant change at the end of the administration period. Therefore, the direction of recovery is determined and only selected dose groups are considered. One-sided tests in the "opposite direction" are appropriate, i.e. a proof of non-inferiority can be recommended. Notice, the phrase *non-inferiority* is used for efficacy endpoints in randomized clinical trials; see e.g., [66]. Both tests on equivalence or tests on non inferiority need the *a priori* definition of still tolerable thresholds. However, these thresholds are commonly not available in toxicology. Therefore, the estimation of $(1 - 2\alpha)$ confidence intervals (claiming equivalence) or $(1 - \alpha)$ confidence intervals (claiming non-inferiority) for comparisons of the dose group against control can be used with their *posthoc* interpretation of what amount is tolerable.

As an example, body weight data of the sub-chronic gavage study on riddelline in female F344 rats are used for a control and four doses [6]. We simplify the data using final weights for the administration period at week 14 for all randomized rats and for the recovery period at week 28 body weights of only 5 rats; see the raw data in Table 2.26.

```
> data("recov", package="SiTuR")
> riddR <-recov[, c(1,4,19 ,33)]
> colnames(riddR) <-c("AnimalNo", "Dose", "w14", "w28")
> riddC <-riddR[is.na(riddR$w28)==FALSE, ]
```

First, the final body weights of the administration period alone are analyzed by a Dunnett procedure in order to identify which dose groups are changed with respect to control and in which direction.

```
> library("multcomp")
> ridd14 <-riddO[riddO$Time=="w14",]
> modRidd <-lm(Bodyweight~Dose, data=ridd14)
> pvalRidd <-summary(glht(modRidd, linfct=mcp(Dose="Dunnett")))
```

For Dose 3 and Dose 4 significant body weight retardation can be stated ($p_{D3-C} = 0.022$, $p_{D4-C} = 0.002$). For these two doses the reversibility after recovery period will be investigated.

The boxplots for the dose-by-time-interaction in Figure 2.20 show a recovery effect, i.e. a monotone decreasing dose-response relationship for the treatment data (w14) (lower boxes)

Table 2.26: Recovery Period Data of Riddelline Bioassay

AnimalNo	Dose	Time	Bodyweight
22	C	w14	237.9
24	C	w14	218.4
26	C	w14	211.8
29	C	w14	226.0
37	C	w14	231.9
...	...	...	...
181	D4	w28	218.8
183	D4	w28	219.4
189	D4	w28	238.2
195	D4	w28	225.0
200	D4	w28	184.6

and a shifted monotone relationship for the recovery week (w28) (upper boxes). However, these dose-relationships seem to be not parallel, i.e., a quantitative interaction may exist. Because the same animal was weighed at week 14 and week 28, a paired design exists for this repeated measures multiple doses design. Therefore a mixed effect model is used for the interaction factor dose-by-time (denoted as IA) with a related random term random=~1/AnimalNo assuming a random intercept. The interaction contrast approach (see Section 2.4.1) interpret differences between week 28 and week 14 for the differences between the dose groups and the control, roughly spoken difference of differences.

```
> library("nlme")
> mixM <- lme(Bodyweight ~ IA-1, data=riddO, random=~1|AnimalNo)
> riddCI <-confint(glht(mixM, linfct=iaRidd$cmab, df=mixM$fixDF$terms,
+                       alternative="greater"))
```

Table 2.27: Interaction Contrasts for Recovery vs. Treatment Period

	Effect size	Lower confidence limit
((D1 - C):w28) - ((D1 - C):w14)	4.62	-8.36
((D2 - C):w28) - ((D2 - C):w14)	8.36	-4.62
((D3 - C):w28) - ((D3 - C):w14)	2.20	-10.78
((D4 - C):w28) - ((D4 - C):w14)	-3.32	-16.30

In Table 2.27 the point estimators (effect sizes) of the differences of differences are presented together with their 95% simultaneous one-sided lower confidence limits for non-inferiority (where body weight retardation is regarded as an effect after the administration period). A positive point estimator tells us that for this dose gradient a recovery effect exists. This effect would be significant if a positive lower limit existed. If we tolerated a 5 g smaller body weight gradient, we would claim a tolerable recovery only for dose D2 with respect to control (i.e. the confidence limit is −4.6). Confidence intervals for ratios in the two-sample paired design are available [291].

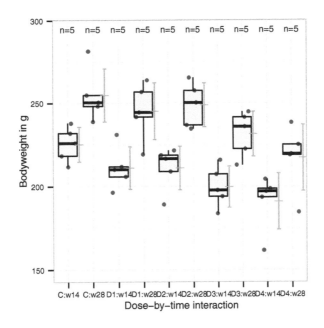

FIGURE 2.20: Boxplots of dose-by-time interactions.

```
> library("pairedCI")
> ridd4 <-ridd0[ridd0$Dose=="D4", ]
> admin <-ridd4[ridd4$Time=="w14",]
> recov <-ridd4[ridd4$Time=="w28",]
> pair <-paired.Loc(admin$Bodyweight,recov$Bodyweight, method="parametric",
+                   alternative="greater")
```

By means of the package `pairedCI` the ratio estimate $Bodyweight_{admin}/Bodyweight_{recov}$ was estimated to 0.879 and the upper 95% confidence limit 0.858, i.e. reversibility can be assumed if we tolerate about 85% of the body weight.

2.2   Trend tests

2.2.1   Aims and limitations

Trend tests (or more precisely tests for ordered alternatives) are highly relevant in toxicology because of two major items: i) a design with a zero dose and several dose levels is used as standard, and ii) claiming a trend belongs to the causation criteria for most of the assays.

We distinguish models and significance tests to claim a trend [363]. Models are usually used for concentrations (instead of doses) with a large(r) number of concentrations and aiming parameter estimation, such as the IC_{50} or benchmark dose. For details see Section 7. In contrast, significance tests are commonly used either only with few doses, aiming at global trend detection or detection of a selected dose, such as maximum safe dose. It is important how the dose levels are considered only, as ordered categories like in contrast tests or as a quantitative covariate like in regression-type tests. Transforming the dose levels $[0, 10, 50, 100 mg/kg]$ into the categories $[control, low, medium, high]$ seems to be an unacceptable loss of information. Well, it depends on the context. If the relationship between dose and concentration at the target tissue is complicated non-linearly and the selection of an appropriate specific dose-concentration model function is difficult, the trend test can be a good choice. Therefore, the guidelines recommend either the use of a trend test (without a specification) or particularly the Williams- trend test (as in the US NTP [9]).

A further classification is the claim for only a global trend, or for a specific dose, such as minimum significant dose (proof of hazard) or maximal safe dose (proof of safety), again under order restriction. The minimum significant dose can be determined using the closed testing procedure; see Section 2.2.2. Somewhat related is also information on the shape of the dose-response relationship, i.e. convex, concave, linear.

Ordered inference can be formulated by a global null hypothesis $H_0 : \mu_0 = \mu_1 = ... = \mu_k$ versus a global order restricted alternative $H_A : \mu_0 \leq \mu_1 \leq .... \leq \mu_k$ with at least one strict inequality (or any pattern of equalities and inequalities up to completely inequalities $\mu_0 < \mu_1 < ... < \mu_k$). The consequence is that both extreme shapes represent a trend in the same way: $H_A^1 : \mu_0 = \mu_1 = ... = \mu_{k-1} < \mu_k$ and $H_A^2 : \mu_0 < \mu_1 = ... = \mu_k$, that are hard to accept by some toxicologists as *trend*. Moreover, some believe a linear trend is the *natural* trend. This is not the case; it rather is a very specific situation, hard to select because of the many equally competing trend alternatives.

Two objectives are responsible for choosing a trend test: i) the use as a causation criterion and ii) the aim to increase the power (compared to tests with unrestricted alternatives). The first usually is under-, and the second mostly overrated. For example, for a four-group design with the expected values 0, 0, 1, 3 ($n_i = 10, SD = 2.2$) the any-pair power of the one-sided Dunnett-test is 0.82 whereas for the trend-type Williams-test it is 0.88.

```
> library("MCPAN")
> muE <-c(0,0,1,3)
> powDu <-powermcpt(mu=muE, n=c(10,10,10,10), sd=2.2, type = "Dunnett",
+   alternative ="greater", ptype = "anypair")
> powWi <-powermcpt(mu=muE, n=c(10,10,10,10), sd=2.2, type = "Williams",
+   alternative ="greater", ptype = "anypair")
```

Two different forms of trend test statistics can be distinguished: i) the quadratic form based on maximum-likelihood estimates under order restriction

$$E_k^2 = \frac{\sum_{i=0}^{k} n_i (\hat{\mu}_i - \bar{X}_{..})^2}{\sum_{i=0}^{k} \sum_{j=1}^{n_i} (X_{ij} - \bar{X}_{..})^2}$$

[36] (where the MLE $\hat{\mu}_i$ are the group means $\bar{X}_i$ when monotone ordered or weighted averaged means satisfying order restriction) or ii) max-type of linear forms: the multiple contrast test $T_{max} = max(T_1, ..., T_\zeta)$ (with $T_l = \frac{\sum_{i=0}^{k} c_{li} \bar{X}_i}{s \sqrt{\sum_{i=0}^{k} c_{li}^2 / n_i}}$, and ζ number of chosen contrasts).

The advantage of the E_k^2-test is its power optimality for any shape, its disadvantage is the complicated distribution (particularly under the alternative) and the non-availability of simultaneous confidence intervals. The advantage of the T_{max}-test is the availability of simultaneous confidence intervals and the distribution even under the alternative, its disadvantage is the apparent arbitrariness of the contrast matrix which leads to various test variations, i.e. Williams-type [400], Marcus-type [254], isotone-type [175], changepoint-type [160], and so on. A permutation-based version of E_k^2-test is available in the package

IsoGene for a matrix of endpoints, denoted as Probe.ID. A toy example with ten non-significant (ps1), ten monotone increasing (ps2), and ten non-monotone gene-probe sets (ps3) is used in a design with control, low and high dose, and three replicates each.

```
> library("IsoGene")
> set.seed(17051949)
> doses <- c(rep(1,3),rep(2,3),rep(3,3))
> ps1 <- matrix(rnorm(90, 1,1),10,9)  # 10 genes with no trends
> ps2 <- matrix(c(rnorm(30, 1,1), rnorm(30,2,1),
+                 rnorm(30,4,1)), 10, 9)  # 10 genes with incr. trends
> ps3 <- matrix(c(rnorm(30, 4,1), rnorm(30,1,1),
+                 rnorm(30,2,1)), 10, 9)  # 10 genes without trends
> probeset <- data.frame(rbind(ps1, ps2,ps3))
> rp <- IsoRawp(doses, probeset, niter = 100)
> pvalE2 <-rp$rawp.up[, 1:3]
```

The one-sided p-values for an increasing trend for the E_k^2-test (abbreviated E2) and the Williams test are reported in Table 2.28.

Table 2.28: Bartholomew (E2) and Williams Tests: One-Sided Adjusted p-Values

Probe.ID	E2	Williams
1	0.26	0.21
2	0.68	0.91
3	0.34	0.32
4	0.61	0.57
5	0.21	0.19
6	0.82	0.97
7	0.33	0.29
8	0.11	0.13
9	0.14	0.19
10	0.63	0.70
11	0.00	0.00
12	0.00	0.00
13	0.02	0.02
14	0.02	0.02
15	0.00	0.00
16	0.03	0.03
17	0.00	0.04
18	0.00	0.00
19	0.00	0.00
20	0.00	0.00
21	0.70	0.98
22	0.79	1.00
23	0.70	0.99
24	0.81	1.00
25	0.78	0.99
26	0.68	0.99
27	0.65	0.99
28	0.62	0.97
29	0.66	0.98
30	0.67	0.88

As expected, the p-values for the first and last 10 probe sets are large, whereas those of probe sets 11–20 are rather small. A consideration of the advantages and disadvantages of the E_k^2-test compared to the Williams-test [169] results in the recommendation of Williams-type tests. In some toxicological assays a downturn effect at high doses is likely (see Section 2.1.2.2 for details), i.e. a non-monotonic dose-response relationship occurs. Tests without any order restriction, such as Dunnett test, seem to be the only way. Although an initial trend is present, no trend claim is possible using such a Dunnett-type approach. A way out is the downturn-protected trend test claiming an initial trend; see Section 2.2.2.

2.2.1.0.1 Trend test or non-linear model? To assume dose as a qualitative factor or a quantitative covariate result in quite different approaches: trend tests (see Section 2.2), or non-linear models (see e.g. Section 7). Various conditions determine usually these methods choice. For example, very few dose levels rather suggest a trend test, while the aim of an low-dose extrapolation suggest a particular non-linear model. This creates the impression that trend test and non-linear models are completely separate approaches. Not necessarily!

Consider a simple one-way layout with 3 dose levels, as occurs for example in genetic association studies; see Section 2.1.5. The contrast for the additive mode of inheritance shows little power. A test with the contrast coefficient (-1,0,1) ignores simply the heterozygous level. By contrast, the linear regression model reveals a higher power. On the other hand, the contrast test for the dominant mode of inheritance reveals high power because the contrast test with (-1, 0.5,0.5) is superior to the regression model. Therefore there is a need to combine both concepts. The extension of the maximum test on three regression models for the arithmetic, ordinal, and logarithmic-linear dose metameters [380]. by means of multiple marginal models [307] (see further details in Section 5.4) can be used to include both regression models and a multiple contrast test. As an example the lung weight data are used again (see the raw data in Table 2.2 and the boxplots in Figure 2.3 in Section 2.1.2). Four marginal models are needed: three regression models for arithmetic(sN), ordinal(sO) and log-linear(SLL) dose metameters and the ANOVA model with the factor dose. Table 2.29 shows the multiplicity adjusted p-values for these 4 models where the regression model with the arithmetic dose scores $|0, 5, 10, 20, 40|$ reveals the smallest p-value; see 2016.

```
> library("multcomp")
> library("ggplot2")
> library("xtable")
> data("acryl", package="SiTuR")
>     Dlevels<-as.numeric(levels(acryl$dose))
>     SO<-log(Dlevels[2])-log(Dlevels[3]/Dlevels[2])*(Dlevels[2]-Dlevels[1])/
+       (Dlevels[3]-Dlevels[2])
>     acryl$DoseN<-as.numeric(as.character(acryl$dose))
>     acryl$DoseO<-as.numeric(acryl$dose)
>     acryl$DoseL<-log(acryl$DoseN)
>     acryl$DoseLL< acryl$DoseL; acryl$DoseLL[acryl$DoseN==Dlevels[1]] <-SO
>     sN <-lm(LungWt~DoseN, data=acryl)
>     sO <-lm(LungWt~DoseO, data=acryl)
>     sLL <-lm(LungWt~DoseLL, data=acryl)
>     lmW<-lm(LungWt~dose, data=acryl) # linear model with factor dose
> TUWI<- glht(mmm(covariate=sN, ordinal=sO, linlog=sLL, wil=lmW),
+               mlf(covariate="DoseN=0", ordinal="DoseO=0",
```

```
+                    linlog="DoseLL=0",wil=mcp(dose = "Williams")))
> sTUWI <-fortify(summary(TUWI))[, c(1,6)]
> colnames(sTUWI) <-c("Comparison", "$p$-value")
> print(xtable(sTUWI, digits=3, caption="Covariate and factor in a trend test",
+       label="tab:TUWII"), include.rownames=FALSE, caption.placement = "top")
```

Table 2.29: Covariate and Factor in a Trend Test

Comparison	p-value
covariate: DoseN	0.004
ordinal: DoseO	0.020
linlog: DoseLL	0.020
wil: C 1	0.015
wil: C 2	0.105
wil: C 3	0.340
wil: C 4	0.525

2.2.2 Closed testing procedure and order restriction

Closed testing procedures formulate first all interesting elementary hypotheses, followed by all of its intersection hypotheses, up to the global hypothesis. These many hypotheses form a closed under intersection hypotheses system. For a class of elementary hypotheses, such as Dunnett-type comparisons or multiple endpoints, the system forms a complete family, where the intersection hypotheses are particularly simple. A further special case is the assumption of an order restriction with the following logical restriction: whenever a trend test up to dose ϕ is significant, at least $H_A : \mu_0 < \mu_\phi$ holds true irrespective of the lower doses. The closure principle is substantially simplified. For example, if the global hypothesis $H_0 : \mu_C = \mu_l = \mu_m = \mu_h$ can be rejected at level α, we can test the next lower hypothesis $H_0 : \mu_C = \mu_l = \mu_m$, again at level α, etc. The procedure stops when the first non-significant hypothesis is reached (or at the 2 sample comparison). This approach is rather flexible because any level α-test can be used for a particular hypothesis [178].

2.2.3 Trend tests for different endpoint types and different designs

A much greater diversity of trend tests is needed in toxicology for the different endpoint types and design versions: Table 2.30 provides an overview of the different available trend tests under different conditions.

Table 2.30: Types of Trend Tests

Endpoint	Condition	Trend test	Ref	Example assay	Section
Normal-distributed	Homogeneous variances	Williams test	[51]	creatine kinase	2.1.2
	Heterogeneous variances	Williams test using sandwich estimator	[159]	creatine kinase	2.1.2.1
		Williams test using Welch-type df	[146]	creatine kinase	2.1.3.1
	Ratio-to-control	Williams-type test for ratios	[95]	creatine kinase	2.1.3
	Non-monotone shape	downturn protected Williams test	[54]	blood nitrogen urea	2.1.2.2
	Quadratic form	Bartholomew test	[36]	simulated probe sets	2.2
	Dunnett and Williams test	User-defined contrast test	[204]	creatine kinase	
	Using historical control data	Williams-type test	[179]	HET-MN assay	4.10
	Per-litter behavioral data	mixed-model based Williams test		creatine kinase	5.6
Arbitrary-distributed	Rank test	Williams-type test for relative effect sizes	[225]	creatine kinase	2.1.4
Proportions	2-by-k table data	Williams-type test in GLM			2.1.6.3
		Optimal scores CA-test	[177]	droplet degeneration, SHE-assay	2.1.6.2
		CA-test, linear-by-linear association test	[194]	droplet degeneration	2.1.6
		ADD2-Williams-type intervals	[346]	droplet degeneration	2.1.6.4
	Crude tumor rates	ADD1-Williams-type intervals	[188]	NTP588 bioassay	3.3.1
	Using historical tumor rates	ADD1-Williams-type intervals	[215]	bronchial adenomas	3.3.2
	2-by-k table data	Profile l. intervals		bronchiolar tumors	2.1.6.5
	Per animal with possible overdispersion	Williams-type test		*in-vivo* miconucleus assay, number of dead fetuses per number of fetuses	2.1.6.6
	Per animal with possible overdispersion	GEE-based Williams-type test		litter-specific abnormal pup counts	5.3
Tumors	Tumors without cause of death information	poly-k based Williams-type test	[347]	incidence of skin fibromas	3.5
	Incidental tumors	stratified Williams-type test		lung alveolar cell adenoma	3.4.1
	Sex as strata	stratified Williams-type test		beta-picoline bioassay	3.4.1.1
Time-to-event data	Crude tumor rates	Tarone-style permutation Williams-type test		piperonyl butoxide carcinogenicity bioassay	3.2.1
	Survival functions	Cox-model based Williams-type test	[157]	NTP TR-120 bioassay	3.2.2
	With random factors	frailty Cox-model and Williams-test	[157]	Litter-matched time-to-response raw data	3.6.4
Counts	Non-monotone shape	downturn protected Williams test	[54]	TA98 Ames assay	4.2
	Overdispersed, near-to zero	FT-transformed (Dunnett-test)	[179]	HET-MN assay	4.7
Multiple endpoints		Williams-test for ratios-to-control	[144]		
Graded histological findings	Severity scores	Williams-test for relative effects	[225]	hyperplasia in parotid gland	2.1.8
	Collapsed severity scores	Max(Max))-test		liver basophilia severity scores	2.1.8.1
	Severity scores	Umbrella Williams-type test		severity scores of hyaline droplets	2.1.8

2.3 Reference values

An important criterion to distinguish between relevant and non-relevant toxic effects —almost unaffected from previously identified statistical significance (or more consequently non-significance) —is whether the concurrent values are within or without endpoint-specific reference values (alternatively denoted as normal ranges or historical control ranges) [178, 240]. The approach seems to be simple: data are collected from q historical controls; these are summarized in a single record of value y_j with a total sample size η. Then an interval is calculated, usually the 2σ-interval $\bar{y}_i \pm 2SD$ or the nonparametric [5%; 95%] percentile interval (here denoted as simplistic), e.g., for red blood count (RBC) $[7.59 - 8.60]$ [64]. This interval is used for toxicological classification e.g., *"...since all of these values were within the respective historical control ranges, all alterations were assessed as incidental and not treatment-related"* [64]. Because this method can relativize the predictive value of the previous statistical tests, caution is advised.

The first question is *which type of interval* should be used from a statistical perspective. Deceptively most intervals for a normally distributed endpoint look similar: $\bar{y}_i \pm k * SD$. However, the factor k (and the specific estimated variance SD) are quite different whether using a confidence interval, a tolerance interval, or a prediction interval. A *confidence interval* contains the population mean of a concurrent population with a pre-specified confidence probability. A *tolerance interval* contains a specified proportion of future samples (with a pre-specified confidence probability), where the number of future samples is not specified. A *prediction interval* contains a single future observation within n future samples, with a pre-specified confidence probability [140]. It seems to be clear that the confidence interval is inappropriate in this context, and the tolerance intervals suffer from a suitable choice of the proportion (90% or 50%) in future samples, whereas the prediction interval seems to be appropriate for toxicological reasoning. A certain interval from historical controls of size η is estimated in such a way that a single future value in either concurrent dose group is within the interval. In such a case a significant effect can be assessed as incidental, otherwise as treatment-related (vice versa). Instead of a prediction interval for a future single value, alternatively a prediction interval for a future mean (of size n_i) can be estimated [140]. Such an interval also depends on n_i, which seems to be useful for regulatory studies with recommended sample sizes.

The second question is *which value*: the group mean, or an individual value within a group or the difference to control (as formulated by [240]: *"A difference ... to control... is less likely to be an effect of treatment if ... it is within ... the range of historical control values..."*. A difference-to-control prediction interval is hard to imagine, but a prediction interval for either a single future value or a group mean value (of sample size n) is possible, but they are quite different. The above mentioned factor k is $t_{df=\eta-1,1-\alpha/2}\sqrt{1/\eta + 1/n}$ and depends on the sample size of the historical controls η as well as the sample size of the future mean n. For predicting a single future value the special case $n = 1$ applies, whereas for the prediction of a mean its sample size $n > 1$ matters [140]. The difference between the two intervals: i) for a future single value, or ii) for a future group mean is substantial and depends furthermore (slightly) on the size of historical data η; see Table 2.31.

Table 2.31: Factor k for a Prediction Interval for a Single Future Value or a Future Group Mean

η	2σ	single future value	mean of $n_i = 10$	mean of $n_i = 20$
20	2.0	2.14	0.81	0.66
60	2.0	2.02	0.68	0.52
∞	2.0	1.96	0.62	0.44

The common-used 2σ intervals can be used as an approximate prediction interval for not too few historical controls for the prediction of a single future value only (notice, 2σ is an approximation for $z_{1-\alpha/2}\sigma = 1.96 * \sigma$). For prediction of a group mean the 2σ intervals are much too wide, i.e. the classification of the test result into *no treatment related effect* by means of a 2σ interval is dangerously biased in toxicology.

The third question is whether we can ignore the between-assay variability in the historical controls (and also the number q of studies). It seems too obvious to assume some degree of between-assay variability. Can we assume a single data record of size η or should we take the variability between the q historical studies into account? Historical assays can be modeled as a random factor to estimate prediction intervals for random effects models [345]. A simulation study revealing the coverage probability of the simplistic intervals becomes too small with a smaller number of historical studies q as well as smaller samples sizes n_η [345]. Even for $q = 10$ historical studies with size $\eta = 10$ an unacceptable liberal behavior occurs, i.e. the interval is falsely too short. The simplistic intervals can only be suggested for > 20 historical studies with > 20 sample sizes, a strong restriction in regulatory toxicology. For several between to within-study variability ratios and even small q, n_η the random effects model keeps the 95% level and can be suggested. A related R package `mixADA` can be used [339, 343]; see the example below.

The fourth question is whether the type of endpoint is relevant. It is seriously relevant. In contrast to the outcome of the t-test (which is to some extent robust for slightly skewed data), the prediction interval is rather biased, if data are skewed. The percentile interval is a robust nonparametric approach and would be perfect, however, it seems to be not yet available for a random effects model. Therefore, the distribution of continuous endpoints should be at least checked for skewness. For large sample sizes and negligible between–assay variability, tests against normal /log-normal distribution exist. However, if the total sample size is small (i.e. < 100) and the between assay variability cannot be ignored, we need a specific solution. For mixed models the Box –Cox λ parameter can be estimated ($\lambda \Rightarrow 1$ normal distribution, $\lambda \Rightarrow 0$ log-normal distribution) [138]. This will be demonstrated.

The fifth question is whether two-sided intervals instead of directed one-sided limits should be used as standard. Although two-sided intervals are quite common, one-sided limits can be recommended for pathological endpoint types, such as tumor rates. Not surprising, the two-sided intervals are wider, and this leads to a premature decision in favor of *not treatment related*. This may be problematic for directional pathological endpoints, such as tumor rates, where only an increase has a toxicological meaning.

```
> data("HistNC", package="SiTuR")
```

As an example the number of micronuclei (MN) in 25 historical pseudo-assays (runs and assays) is used [179]. The problem with these data is the larger number of zero MN and the count character at all. Therefore, a Freeman–Tukey transformation (see Section 2.1.9) was used; see the boxplot in Figure 2.21.

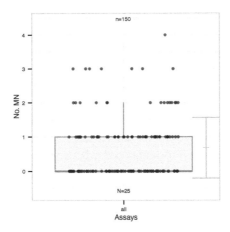

FIGURE 2.21: Number of MN in 25 historical runs.

```
> library("mixADA")
> library("lme4")
> fiNC <-lmer(ftt ~ 1 + (1|run), data=HistNC)
> summary(fiNC)
> fs <-mixADA:::predint_lmer(fit=fiNC, type="h1", level=0.95,
+                            alternative="less")$predint
> predI <-quantile(HistNC$ftt,probs=0.95)
> library("EnvStats")
> pI <-predIntNorm(HistNC$ftt, n.mean = 1)$interval$limits[2]
```

The upper prediction limit in the random effects model is 3.36, for the percentile 3.47 and for the 2σ interval 3.65. When using the random effects model in this micronuclei example, more future values will be declared as potentially problematic compared with the less appropriate methods.

2.4 Analysis of complex designs

The standard design is an one-way layout with the treatment levels: negative control (NC), low dose, medium dose, high dose. More complex designs include:

- higher-way layout, commonly two-way layout, e.g., for the primary factor *treatment* and the secondary factor *sex*

- incomplete designs between one-way and two-way layouts, e.g., using a joint control

- block designs, whereas the common block in toxicology is the cage with several animals

- stratified designs (see details in Section 3.4.1)

- designs with a covariate, i.e., analysis of covariance

- designs with repeated measures

2.4.1 Analysis of interactions: Evaluation of sex by treatment interaction

Commonly, in repeated toxicity studies on rodents animals of both sexes are used. The independent analysis of both sexes is the standard approach whereas this conservative approach can be replaced by two alternatives: i) conditional pooling over the sexes based on ANOVA pre-testing for no-interaction, ii) joint evaluation in a cell means model. A cell means model is a pseudo one-way layout for the factor IA (interaction), generated from the primary factor `dose` and the secondary factor `sex`. Relative liver weight data from a 13-week study on female F344 rats administered with sodium dichromate dihydrate were used [3] as an example.

The interaction test of the ANOVA is significant, but this global test provides no information which dose(s) reveal different patterns.

```
> data("livMF", package="SiTuR")
> livmf <-livMF
> livmf$relLiv <-livmf$LiverWt/livmf$BodyWt
> livmf$relLiv100 <-100*livmf$relLiv # distinguishable sum of squares
> livmf$Dose <-as.factor(livmf$Dose)
> livmf$IA <-livmf$Dose:livmf$Sex
> livMales <-livmf[livmf$Sex=="males", ]
> livFemales <-livmf[livmf$Sex=="females", ]
```

Table 2.32: ANOVA for Global Interaction Test

	Df	Sum Sq	Mean Sq	F value	Pr(>F)
Dose	5	1.07	0.21	5.68	0.0001
Sex	1	1.27	1.27	33.61	0.0000
Dose:Sex	5	0.95	0.19	4.99	0.0004
Residuals	108	4.09	0.04		

The conclusion is the use of separate Dunnett-tests for males and females; see the simultaneous confidence intervals in Figure 2.22.

```
> library("multcomp")
> modM <-lm(relLiv~Dose, data=livMales)
> modF <-lm(relLiv~Dose, data=livFemales)
> plot(glht(modM, linfct=mcp(Dose="Dunnett")), main="Males",
+       xlab="Simultaneous confidence interval")
> plot(glht(modF, linfct=mcp(Dose="Dunnett")), main="Females",
+       xlab="Simultaneous confidence interval")
```

For the interaction factor IA in the cell mean model Dunnett-by-Tukey dose-by-sex interaction contrasts can be estimated [214] to identify at which dose vs. control comparison(s) the interaction occur(s).

```
> library("statint", quietly=TRUE)
> iaDS <-iacontrast(livmf$Dose, livmf$Sex, typea="Dunnett", typeb="Tukey")
> modIA <-lm(relLiv~IA-1, data=livmf)# without intercept
```

```
> library("multcomp")
> sumIA <-summary(glht(modIA, linfct=mcp(IA=iaDS$cmab)))
```

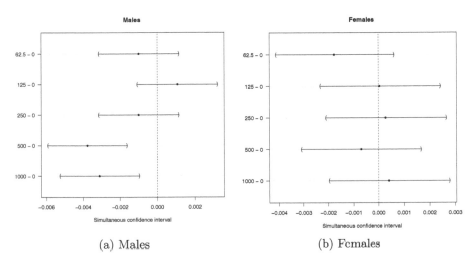

(a) Males   (b) Females

FIGURE 2.22: Sex-specific Dunnett tests for relative liver weight data.

Table 2.33: Interaction Contrasts for Relative Liver Weight Data

Interaction comparisons	Test statistics	p-value
((62.5 - 0):males) - ((62.5 - 0):females)	0.619	0.958
((125 - 0):males) - ((125 - 0):females)	0.836	0.872
((250 - 0):males) - ((250 - 0):females)	-1.044	0.744
((500 - 0):males) - ((500 - 0):females)	-2.484	0.059
((1000 - 0):males) - ((1000 - 0):females)	-2.862	0.022

In Table 2.33 we see significant difference between males and females for the difference of the highest dose against control. In other studies other interactions may be of interest, such as time-by-dose.

2.4.2 Analysis of designs between one- and two-way layouts

There exist designs, looking like one-way layouts, but they are actually incomplete two-way layouts. One example is a drug combination experiment with only one joint control. Raw data are available in the package **drc** for a dose-response relationship of a mixture of alkyl oleates with the herbicide phenmedipham (M) or phenmedipham alone (P) applied to galium aparine [67]. In order to convey the problem better didactically, we selected 3 of 11 doses; see the raw data in Table 2.34 and the boxplots in Figure 2.23 where the factor IAfac represents the interaction term.

```
> data("gaa", package="SiTuR")
```

Table 2.34: Dry Matter Raw Data of Phenmidipham Herbicide on Galium Aparine

Drymatter	Dose	Treatment	InteractionFactor
1146	0	C	0:C
1005	0	C	0:C
756	0	C	0:C
1108	0	C	0:C
956	0	C	0:C
989	0	C	0:C
1109	0	C	0:C
867	0	C	0:C
864	0	C	0:C
997	0	C	0:C
891	0	C	0:C
744	0	C	0:C
...	...	...	
498	100	M	100:M
471	100	M	100:M
565	100	M	100:M
635	100	M	100:M
302	200	M	200:M
268	200	M	200:M
302	200	M	200:M
481	200	M	200:M
331	200	M	200:M
291	200	M	200:M
292	200	M	200:M
315	200	M	200:M
313	200	M	200:M
291	200	M	200:M

The analysis of such complex designs by means of user-defined specifically defined multiple contrast tests is described [348]. In our example six specific contrasts are defined (in the contrast matrix `contrIA`): comparison vs. control for all groups, comparison of the mixture (M) vs. the herbicide alone (P) for all doses, the comparison of the low dose vs. 100 and vs. 200 (for both formulations), and the dose-by-treatment interactions for 100 vs. 12 and 200 vs. 12. (Notice more comparisons could be formulated.) In Figure 2.24 the upper simultaneous confidence limits for theses contrasts can be seen. It shows: i) a significant decrease vs. all groups, ii) a slight decrease of Mix vs. P, iii) a clear decrease of 100 vs. 12 and even a stronger one of 200 vs. 12 , iv) a non-significant interaction for 100 vs. 12 but a significant interaction for 200 vs 12, i.e., Mix behaves differently in comparison to P at 200 compared with 12.

```
> library("multcomp")
> data("gaa", package="SiTuR")
> gaaM <-lm(drymatter~IAfac-1, data=gaa)
> contrIA <- rbind("All vs. C" = c(-1, 1/6, 1/6, 1/6, 1/6, 1/6, 1/6),
+          "Mix vs. P" = c(0, -1/3, 1/3, -1/3, 1/3, -1/3, 1/3),
+          "100 vs. 12" = c(0, -1/2, -1/2, 1/2, 1/2, 0, 0),
+          "200 vs. 12" = c(0, -1/2, -1/2, 0, 0, 1/2, 1/2),
+          "Interact Mix vs. \n  100 vs 12" = c(0, 1, -1, -1, 1, 0, 0),
+          "Interact Mix vs. \n  200 vs 12" = c(0, 1, -1, 0, 0, -1, 1))
> par(mar=c(4,7,2,2))
```

```
> plot(glht(gaaM, linfct=mcp(IAfac=contrIA), alternative="less"), main="",
+      xlab="",cex.axis=0.6, cex.main=0.6)
```

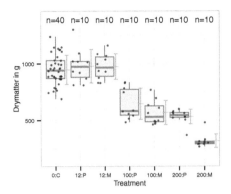

FIGURE 2.23: Boxplots for dose-by-treatment interactions.

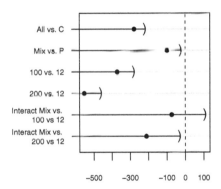

FIGURE 2.24: Simultaneous confidence limits for interaction contrasts.

Because of the high correlation between these contrasts, such a detailed analysis is not too conservative.

2.4.3 Analysis of block designs

A block is a non-randomized secondary factor, such as cage. By defining a block with certain levels, a measurable (e.g., initial body weight) or non-measurable (e.g., analyst) nuisance factor can be controlled. This block factor is not subject of inference (neither in a global F-test nor multiple comparisons between its levels) and it cannot be used to test interactions to the primary factor (e.g., dose). Its objective is to explain a certain amount of variability and therefore to reduce the residual error.

As an example the body weight data of a two-year bioassay on mercuric chloride were used [4]. Five female rats were caged together, and therefore in each of the treatment groups (control, 2.5, and 5 mg/ml MeCl) 12 cages were used yielding an initial sample size of 60 per group. For demonstration purposes, the body weight at week 13 was used, adjusted for ratio-to-baseline (with the baseline being the body weight at week 1); see the raw data in Table 2.35.

```
> data("mercur", package="SiTuR")
> mercur$Cage <- as.factor(mercur$Cage)
> mercur$Animal <- as.factor(mercur$Animal)
> mercur$Dose <- factor(mercur$Dose,
+                 levels=c("Vehicle Control", "2.5 mg/kg", "5 mg/kg"))
> mercur$Bodywt13 <-as.numeric(mercur$Week.13)/as.numeric(mercur$Week.1)
> merc <-na.omit(droplevels(mercur[, c(1,2,3,10)]))
```

Table 2.35: Raw Data of Cage-Specific Body Weights at Week 13

Animal	Cage	Dose	Bodywt13
30233	13	Vehicle Control	5.05
30234	13	Vehicle Control	1.18
30235	13	Vehicle Control	1.09
30236	13	Vehicle Control	2.35
30237	13	Vehicle Control	1.51
...	...	...	...
30528	72	5 mg/kg	0.91
30529	72	5 mg/kg	0.77
30530	72	5 mg/kg	0.61
30531	72	5 mg/kg	0.36
30532	72	5 mg/kg	0.67

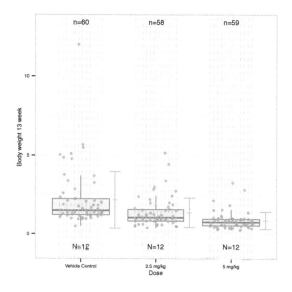

FIGURE 2.25: Boxplots for cage-specific body weights (ratios to baseline) at week 13.

Notice, a block design assumes the random treatment allocation with each pre-defined cage. If the cages are randomly assigned to treatments and the responses are measured on multiple units within each cage a subsampling problem exists which can be analyzed by a mixed effect model (see Section 5.2). The boxplots in Figure 2.25 show heterogeneous variances and not necessarily symmetric distributed data. Still, a mixed-effects model using the random factor cage is used in comparison with a linear model without the cage effect.

```
> library("nlme")
> library("multcomp")
> m1 <-lm(Bodywt13 ~ Dose, data=merc)
> mm1 <- lme(Bodywt13 ~ Dose, random=~1|Cage , data=merc)
> dfMM <-anova(mm1)$denDF[2]
> pDm <-summary(glht(m1,linfct = mcp(Dose = "Dunnett")))$test$pvalue[1]
> pDmm <-summary(glht(mm1,linfct = mcp(Dose = "Dunnett"),
+                    df=dfMM))$test$pvalue[1]
```

The p-value for the comparison of low dose vs. control is 7.75×10^{-4} for a linear model (ignoring the cage effect) whereas 0.001918 for a linear mixed-effects model including the random factor cage. It is data-specific that the p-value from the mixed-effects model is larger. In general, a mixed effect model should be used for data with blocks. A simple alternative is the use of block mean transformed data as long as the number of sub-units (i.e., animals within the cage) is nearly balanced, as in the above example.

2.4.4 Analysis of covariance: Evaluation of organ weights

Commonly, the analysis of covariance is used in randomized studies to adjust against subject-specific covariates, such as age and body weight or pre-treatment covariates [354]. Examples in toxicology are the adjustment of organ weights by body weights [207] or pub weights by litter sizes (see Section 5.2). The analysis of organ weights is recommended as an important part of the risk assessment [261, 353]. Relative organ weights are commonly analyzed, e.g., nonparametrically [406]. For an unbiased analysis the dependency between body and organ weight must be linear and the linear regression fit must go through the origin [84], which may be problematic in real data conditions. Because of the possible complex relationship between organ and body weight multivariate methods were proposed [30] and therefore a a bivariate ANOVA-type approach was used here as well.

As an example the liver weights from a 13-week study on female F344 rats administered with sodium dichromate dihydrate were used [3] (see the raw data in Table 2.36) and are analyzed together with the body weights. For the analysis of covariance the standardized body weights adjBodyWt are used as covariate, i.e., the difference of individual body weights to the total mean body weight to achieve the adjustment against the population mean. The question arises whether a dose-related liver weight effect is caused either by being directly affected in the liver, indirectly via changes of body weights, or both. In Figure 2.26 the boxplots for both organ and body weight indicate a retardation at the high doses.

```
> data("liv", package="SiTuR")
> liv$Dose <- as.factor(liv$Dose)
> liv$relLiv <-liv$LiverWt/liv$BodyWt
> liv$adjBodyWt <-liv$BodyWt-mean(liv$BodyWt)
```

Table 2.36: Body and Liver Weight Data

Dose	BodyWt	LiverWt	relLiv	adjBodyWt
0	338	11	0	16
0	319	10	0	-3
0	369	13	0	47
0	373	13	0	51
0	315	10	0	-7
...	...	...	...	...
1000	294	9	0	-28
1000	294	9	0	-28
1000	281	8	0	-41
1000	317	9	0	-5
1000	292	8	0	-30

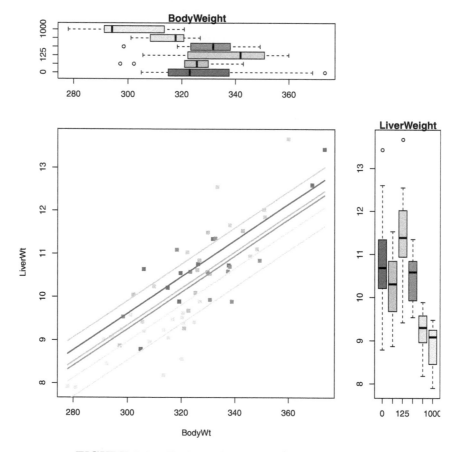

FIGURE 2.26: Body and liver weight data example.

However, the treatment effect may induce changes in organ weight or in body weight or both. Such effects may be proportional between body and organ weight, or not. Such effects may violate the independence assumption in the analysis of covariance [355]. By means of three virtual data conditions this delicate problem will be highlighted and it will be demonstrated that the two proposed methods: relative organ weight and covariance-adjusted organ weight can fail. A multivariate alternative will be proposed, that is a Dunnett-type approach which allows dose-specific claims (not just global ones).

In a first case (i) both a dose-related organ weight (ow) and body weight (bw) retardation occurs whereupon organ and body weight are completely proportional; see both boxplots and prediction for the ANCOVA in the middle panel in Figure 2.27.

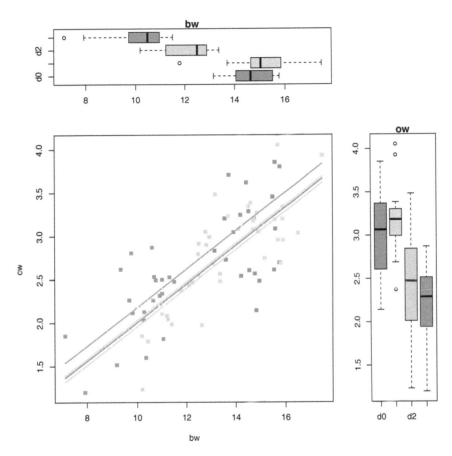

FIGURE 2.27: Proportional organ and body weight retardation.

In case i) pattern, neither global ANOVA-type p-values for relative organ weight (0.3144) nor the ANCOVA-adjustment (0.5001) are significant, whereas they are highly significant for absolute organ weight (p<0.001) (and of course for body weight (p<0.001)). Alternatively, the p-value for the bivariate ANOVA (p<0.001) indicates significant organ and/or body weight effects. This proportionality pattern reveals the problematic evaluation of relative organ weights.

In the second case (ii) we assume an organ weight retardation only, i.e., body weights are unaffected by the treatment; see Figure 2.28.

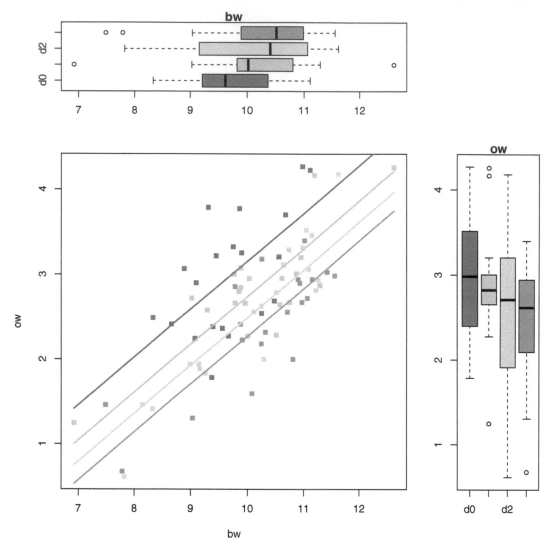

FIGURE 2.28: Organ retardation only.

In case ii) pattern, the global ANOVA-type p values for absolute organ weight is per defi-nition small (0.055), but just not significant, whereas the body weight (0.37)) are not sig-nificant per definition as well. Here, both the global ANCOVA-adjusted analysis (p<0.001) and the relative organ weights are significant (p<0.001), due to the variance reduction by considering a ratio or a covariate. The p-value for the bivariate ANOVA (p<0.001) indicates again significant organ and/or body weight effects.

The third case (iii) is even more complicated but still realistic because only in the highest dose group an increasing organ weight exists, whereas body weight is decreased at the high dose; see Figure 2.29.

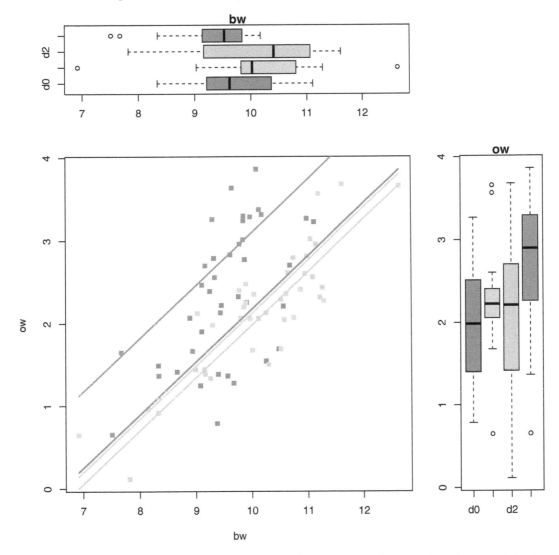

FIGURE 2.29: Treatment effect only at high dose: Increased organ but decreased body weight.

In case iii) pattern all p-values from ANOVA-type analysis are significant, but of a rather different magnitude: for absolute organ weight (0.023), body weight (0.029)), whereas for ANCOVA-adjusted ($p<0.001$), relative organ weights ($p<0.001$), and bivariate ANOVA ($p<0.001$). Both ANCOVA and relative organ weights identify the shifts of the high dose effect more clearly. From these three toy examples it can be concluded, that neither relative organ weights nor analysis of covariance can be recommended as a general approach. In order to identify an effect that occurs only at the high dose the related Dunnett-type comparisons are needed.

Using two-sided Dunnett procedures for comparison of the high dose against control all p-values are significant (again of a different magnitude): absolute organ weight (0.016), ANCOVA-adjusted ($p<0.001$), and relative organ weights ($p<0.001$). In each example the bivariate analysis identified the underlying effects, however this global test allows neither statement which doses are changed nor whether organ weight, body weight, or both are affected. Below a related multivariate Dunnett-type approach will be proposed. The above-discussed detailed analysis will now be performed for the already-mentioned liver weight example. In Figure 2.30 we see first some proportionality between initially increasing followed by decreasing liver weights and body weights. From the second phenomenon, a non-monotone dose response pattern of both liver and body weight, the inappropriateness of global ANOVA (ANCOVA) tests can be guessed. A two-sided Dunnett-type analysis can be recommended in such a case. A bivariate procedure using endpoint-specific linear models and derive the correlations between test statistics through asymptotic arguments [307] using the function mmm in the R package multcomp.

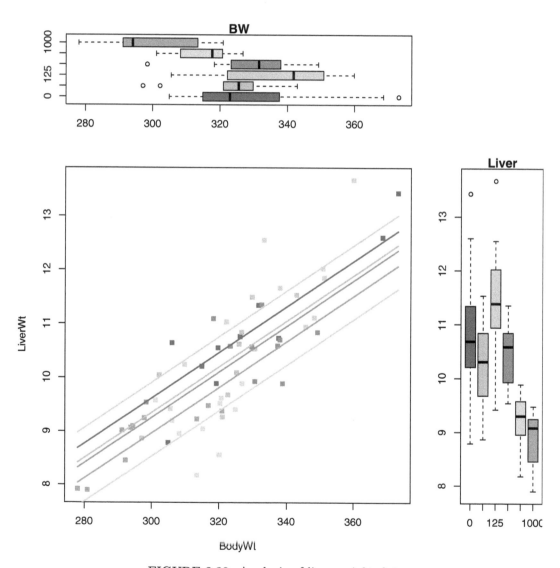

FIGURE 2.30: Analysis of liver weight data.

The fact that all *p*-values of the global tests are significant, namely for absolute liver weight (p<0.001), for body weight (0.001), for ANCOVA-adjusted (p<0.001), for relative liver weights (p<0.001), and for the bivariate ANOVA (p<0.001), is not a counterargument against the use of the multivariate Dunnett-type procedure below. The effect of liver and body weight is simply very large.

```
> library("multcomp")
> library("ggplot2")
> pCOVAR8 <-fortify(summary(glht(fancova, mcp(dose="Dunnett"))))
> prel8 <-fortify(summary(glht(lm(LiverWt/BodyWt~dose, data=liv),
+                     mcp(dose="Dunnett"))))
> pliv8 <-fortify(summary(glht(lm(LiverWt~dose, data=liv),
+                     mcp(dose="Dunnett"))))
> pbw8 <-fortify(summary(glht(lm(BodyWt~dose, data=liv),
+                     mcp(dose="Dunnett"))))

> library("nparcomp")
> pvalNP <-nparcomp(relLiv~dose, data=liv, type="Dunnett",
+          asy.method = "mult.t", plot.simci =FALSE, info = FALSE,
+          correlation=FALSE)$Analysis$p.Value
```

Table 2.37: Five Dunnett-Type Tests for Liver and Body Weight Data

Comp	t_{COVAR}	p_{COVAR}	t_{RelWt}	p_{RelWt}	t_{Liv}	p_{Liv}	t_{Body}	p_{Body}	p_{Nonp}
62.5 - 0	-1.00	0.78	-1.21	0.63	-1.48	0.44	-1.08	0.72	0.85
125 - 0	1.09	0.72	1.29	0.57	1.38	0.51	0.86	0.86	0.80
250 - 0	-1.36	0.53	-1.22	0.62	-0.96	0.80	-0.08	1.00	0.56
500 - 0	-3.94	0.00	-4.56	0.00	-4.21	0.00	-2.01	0.18	0.00
1000 - 0	-2.09	0.15	-3.77	0.00	-5.00	0.00	-4.46	0.00	0.00

In Table 2.37 the effect sizes (e.g., tRelWt) and the related Dunnett-type multiplicity-adjusted *p*-values are shown: covariance-adjusted (COVAR), relative organ weight (RelWt), absolute liver weights (Liv, body weight (Body), and nonparametric evaluation of relative liver weight (Nonp). We see non-significant increased liver and body weights for low doses (by the positive sign of the estimates) and liver and body weight retardation (negative sign) for the 500 and 1000 mg/kg doses. Notice, the high dose is not significant for COVAR.

A bivariate Dunnett-type approach can be achieved by considering two endpoint-specific linear models (mLiv,mBody) where the correlations between these two test statistics is available through asymptotic arguments by the function mmm [307].

```
> library("multcomp")
> mLiv <-lm(LiverWt~Dose, data=liv)
> mBody <-lm(BodyWt~Dose, data=liv)
> mLB <- glht(mmm(LiverWt = mLiv, BodyWt= mBody),
+          mlf(mcp(Dose ="Dunnett")))
```

Table 2.38 shows these multiplicity-adjusted *p*-values of the bivariate Dunnett-type test concluding liver weight retardation (negative sign of estimate) for the 500 and 1000 mg/kg dose and body weight retardation for the high dose only.

This bivariate approach, including a selected organ weight and body weight can be extended to all organ weights and the body weight, as shown for the above example including thymus,

Table 2.38: Bivariate Multiple Comparison of Liver and Body Weight Data

Comparison	Effect size	p-value
LiverWt: 62.5 - 0	-1.482	0.434
LiverWt: 125 - 0	1.378	0.504
LiverWt: 250 - 0	-0.958	0.807
LiverWt: 500 - 0	-4.213	0.000
LiverWt: 1000 - 0	-4.997	0.000
BodyWt: 62.5 - 0	-1.081	0.719
BodyWt: 125 - 0	0.863	0.868
BodyWt: 250 - 0	-0.083	1.000
BodyWt: 500 - 0	-2.012	0.174
BodyWt: 1000 - 0	-4.464	0.000

spleen, heart and liver weights (data selected from a 13-week study on female F344 rats administered with sodium dichromate dihydrate [3]) (see the raw data in Table 2.39).

```
> data("statorgans", package="SiTuR")
```

Table 2.39: Multiple Organ Weight Data

dose	BodyWt	Heart	Liver	Lung	Spleen	Thymus
0.00	337.60	0.89	10.73	1.35	0.69	0.26
0.00	319.20	0.84	9.89	1.25	0.66	0.20
0.00	368.70	0.98	12.60	1.50	0.74	0.22
0.00	373.30	0.97	13.43	1.60	0.69	0.24
0.00	314.90	0.86	10.21	1.19	0.59	0.21
...	...	...	...	...		
1000.00	293.80	0.84	9.07	1.08	0.59	0.21
1000.00	294.40	0.82	9.10	1.16	0.60	0.21
1000.00	280.90	0.66	7.90	1.00	0.56	0.15
1000.00	316.80	0.93	9.48	1.13	0.63	0.21
1000.00	292.20	0.86	8.46	1.21	0.61	0.20

```
> library("multcomp")
> statorgans$Dose <-as.factor(statorgans$dose)
> MTt <-lm(Thymus~Dose, data=statorgans)
> MS <-lm(Spleen~Dose, data=statorgans)
> MLi <-lm(Liver~Dose, data=statorgans)
> MH <-lm(Heart~Dose, data=statorgans)
> MB <-lm(BodyWt~Dose, data=statorgans)
> mORG  <- glht(mmm(Liver = MLi,Heart=MH, Spleen=MS, Thymus=MTt, BodyWt=MB),
+               mlf(mcp(Dose ="Dunnett")))
```

The adjusted p-values in Table 2.40 show significant dose-dependent effects for liver, spleen, and body weight.

2.4.5   Repeated measures: Evaluation of body weights

The analysis of body weights is characterized by a repeated measured weight of the same animal and possibly missing values, possibly treatment dependent. An example is the 5 weights per mice (weeks 1, 8, 15, 22, 29) in four dose groups (0, 2, 10, 20, 100 mg/kg)

Table 2.40: Multivariate Multiple Comparisons of Organ and Body Weight Data

Comparison	p-value
Liver: 62.5 - 0	0.801
Liver: 125 - 0	0.864
Liver: 250 - 0	0.991
Liver: 500 - 0	0.001
Liver: 1000 - 0	0.000
Heart: 62.5 - 0	0.054
Heart: 125 - 0	1.000
Heart: 250 - 0	1.000
Heart: 500 - 0	0.369
Heart: 1000 - 0	0.998
Spleen: 62.5 - 0	0.382
Spleen: 125 - 0	0.970
Spleen: 250 - 0	0.383
Spleen: 500 - 0	0.000
Spleen: 1000 - 0	0.416
Thymus: 62.5 - 0	1.000
Thymus: 125 - 0	0.999
Thymus: 250 - 0	0.986
Thymus: 500 - 0	0.408
Thymus: 1000 - 0	0.999
BodyWt: 62.5 - 0	0.974
BodyWt: 125 - 0	0.997
BodyWt: 250 - 0	1.000
BodyWt: 500 - 0	0.412
BodyWt: 1000 - 0	0.000

in an immunotoxicity study on chloramine [5]. The relevant variables in the dataset are `Anino, dose, time, weight`. Summarized data for the group means for the times $1, 8, 15, 22, 29$ weeks and the dose groups are given in Table 2.41.

```
> data("immun", package="SiTuR")
> meandat <- aggregate(weight ~ dose + time, data=immun, mean)
```

For the dose-by-time plot in Figure 2.31 for both individuals and means, first the dose-specific means per animal are estimated into the object `meandat`.

The subject-specific time dependency can be analyzed in the mixed effects model assuming random slopes and intercepts (model modR1) or the simpler model with random intercepts only (modR2). An old-style approach is the repeated measurement ANOVA [164, 165], just an approximation.

```
> library("lme4")
> library("pbkrtest")
> modR1 <-lmer(weight~dose+time+(time|Anino), data=immun)
>      # animal-specific slopes and intercepts
> modR1a <-lmer(weight~time+(time|Anino), data=immun)
>      # animal-specific slopes and intercepts
> dfff <-as.integer(KRmodcomp(modR1, modR1a)$stats$ddf)
>      # degrees of freedom based on Kenward-Roger approximation
> modR2 <-lmer(weight~dose+time+(1|Anino), data=immun)
>      # only intercepts
```

Table 2.41: Group Means for Repeated Body Weight Data

dose	time	weight
0	1	20.86
2	1	20.92
10	1	20.70
20	1	20.93
100	1	20.98
0	8	21.07
2	8	21.32
10	8	21.00
20	8	21.20
100	8	20.88
0	15	22.21
2	15	22.25
10	15	22.27
20	15	22.36
100	15	22.33
0	22	22.96
2	22	23.38
10	22	23.25
20	22	23.29
100	22	23.43
0	29	24.13
2	29	24.54
10	29	24.41
20	29	24.34
100	29	24.22

The model with the smaller AIC value is chosen, i.e., the more complex model (`modR1`). Using this model, the comparisons of the dose groups against the control are performed by the Dunnett-type procedure; see the simultaneous confidence intervals in Figure 2.32 revealing no significant change in body weight.

```
> library("multcomp")
> plot(glht(modR1, linfct=mcp(dose="Dunnett"), df=dfff),
+       main="", xlab=" ")
```

2.4.5.1   Repeated measures: Inference for both treatment and time effects

Questions arise at which times which doses differ from control. In the following, three approaches are shown in which the familywise error rate is controlled both for time and dose comparison [295]. As an example the body weights after 65 and 105 weeks in a long-term study on mercuric chloride [10] is used where after 65 weeks an interim analysis and after 105 the final analysis were performed (see the raw data with the missing pattern in Table 2.43). Therefore, inference on these two specific time points, together with comparisons of the doses against control, is of interest.

Table 2.42: Comparison of Two Models with Different Random Effects Formulations

	Df	AIC	Pr(>Chisq)
modR2	8	2955.60	
modR1	10	2875.20	0.0000

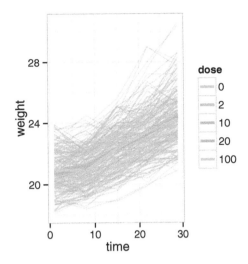

FIGURE 2.31: Body weight time-dependency.

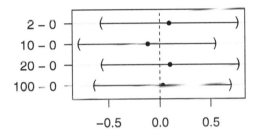

FIGURE 2.32: Simultaneous confidence intervals for body weight data.

```
> data("HgCl", package="SiTuR")
```

Therefore, a related contrast matrix `contDT` is formulated for simultaneous comparisons of dose groups against the control for weeks 65 and 105.

```
> library("multcomp")
> library("plyr")
> library("reshape2")
> HgCl$Cage <- as.factor(HgCl$Cage)
> HgCl$Animal <- as.factor(HgCl$Animal)
> HgCl$Dose <- factor(HgCl$Dose,
+                     levels=c("Vehicle Control", "2.5 mg/kg", "5 mg/kg"))
> mercy <- melt(HgCl, c("Animal", "Cage", "Dose"), variable.name="Week",
+               value.name="Weight")
> dun <- contrMat(numeric(3), "Dunnett")
> contDT <- diag(2)%x%dun
> data65<-subset(mercy, Week=="Week.65")
> data105<-subset(mercy, Week=="Week.105")
> mod065 <- lm(Weight ~ Dose - 1, data=data65,
+              na.action="na.exclude")
> mod105 <- lm(Weight ~ Dose - 1, data105,
```

```
+              na.action="na.exclude")
> MMMDF <- c(mod065$df, mod105$df)
> MercMargMean <- glht(mmm(mod065, mod105),
+              linfct=contDT, df=floor(mean(MMMDF)))
```

Table 2.43: Body Weights after 65 and 105 Weeks

Animal	Cage	Dose	Week.65	Week.105
30233	13	Vehicle Control	307.5	369.2
30234	13	Vehicle Control	284.9	297.9
30235	13	Vehicle Control	313.1	
30236	13	Vehicle Control	300.4	
30237	13	Vehicle Control	308.4	330.8
...	...	...	...	...
30528	72	5 mg/kg		
30529	72	5 mg/kg	262.3	
30530	72	5 mg/kg	270.1	
30531	72	5 mg/kg	271.7	184.6
30532	72	5 mg/kg	250.5	272.0

Table 2.44: Simultaneous Dunnett-Type between Doses and between Times Comparisons

Comparison	Test statistics	p-value
1	-8.15	0.00
2	-9.97	0.00
3	-2.88	0.02
4	-4.31	0.00

All four comparisons of dose against the control for both week 65 and 105 are significant (see Table 2.44).

2.5 Proof of safety

Cases exist where we are interested whether the new drug is harmless or harmless up to a specified dose. The proof of safety should be used with a direct control of the more important false negative error rate [58], [262], whereas the proof of hazard controls the false positive error rate directly (see Section 2.1). The classification of the endpoints for which directed or undirected hypotheses are appropriate is hereby even more important than in the proof of hazard, namely: i) for one-sided hypotheses, tests on non-inferiority are appropriate, whereas ii) for two-sided hypotheses, tests on equivalence. Both for vital sign endpoints (see Section 1.2.3) and pathological findings one-sided confidence intervals for claiming non-inferiority will be demonstrated: the significant toxicity approach for inhibition of *daphnia* offspring [92] and evaluation of tumor rates. Further classifications are the use of independent two-sample test (significant toxicity approach in Section 6) or simultaneous comparisons versus a control, and approaches for difference-to-control or ratio-to-control [111].

2.5.1 One-sided hypotheses: Test on non-inferiority

For a tumor rate, one-sided decisions are appropriate and the following hypotheses are evaluated by non-inferiority tests or related one-sided lower confidence limits

$$H_0 : \pi_i - \pi_0 \leq \delta \text{ harmful}$$
$$H_A : \pi_i - \pi_0 > \delta \text{ harmless}$$

More generally, in the following there are decision rules for one-sided simultaneous confidence limits: i) endpoints where an increase is harmful (e.g., tumor rate): decision in favor of harmlessness if $upperCI_{\mu_i - \mu_0} < \delta$ (or $upperCI_{\mu_i / \mu_0} < \theta$), otherwise harmful (where $\delta > 0; \theta > 1$) or ii) endpoints where a decrease is harmful (e.g., number offsprings): decision in favor of harmlessness if $lowerCI_{\mu_i - \mu_0} > -\delta$ (or $lowerCI_{\mu_i / \mu_0} > 1/\theta$), otherwise harmful.

2.5.1.1 Test of significant toxicity

In whole effluent toxicity assay inhibition of the primary vital endpoint, number of offsprings per live female in *Ceriodaphnia dubia* is of toxicological interest only and therefore the null-hypothesis (assuming the endpoint's expected value μ_i):

$$H_0 : \mu_i / \mu_0 \leq \eta \text{ harmful}$$
$$H_A : \mu_i / \mu_0 > \eta \text{ harmless}$$

is tested by one-sided ratio-to-control tests [337], independent for each concentration. The US EPA defined the tolerable thresholds for acute and chronic assays to: $\eta_{acute} = 0.80$, $\eta_{chronic} = 0.75$. Variance heterogeneity occurs in these reproduction data, namely initially increasing variances with increasing doses but shrinking variances (up to zero) for rather high doses (see e.g., the example below). Therefore, the Welch's type modification [367] was can be recommended as a standard test; see details in Section 6. As an example, the number of young per adult for a control and five concentrations in *daphnia* in a whole effluent toxicity assay is used [12]; see the raw data in Table 2.45.

```
> data("daphnia", package="SiTuR")
```

Table 2.45: Raw Data *Daphnia* Whole Effluent Toxicity Assay

Concentration	Adults	Number_Young
0	1	27
0	2	30
0	3	29
0	4	31
0	5	16
...	...	...
25	6	0
25	7	0
25	8	0
25	9	0
25	10	0

Figure 2.33 shows the related boxplots where an inhibition for higher doses and variance heterogeneity can be seen. The question arises to which dose the test compound is harmless, i.e., reveals an inhibition that is still above the acceptable limit of $\eta = 0.8$.

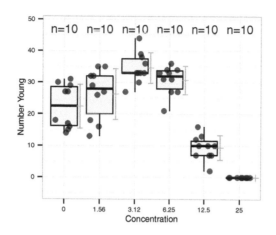

FIGURE 2.33: Boxplot for *Daphnia* data.

A Welch-modified ratio-to-control Dunnett-type test is available in the function `simtest.ratioVH` [95, 146]:

```
> library("mratios")
> daphT <-simtest.ratioVH(Number_Young~conc, data=daphnia,
+                type = "Dunnett", alternative = "less",
+                Margin.vec = rep(0.8,5))$p.value.raw
```

Table 2.46: Adjusted *p*-Values for Ratio-to-Control Non-Inferiority Tests

	p-value
1.56/0	0.9925
3.12/0	1.0000
6.25/0	1.0000
12.5/0	0.0005
25/0	0.0000

The adjusted *p*-values for independent ratio-to-control non-inferiority tests assuming normal distribution, heterogeneous variances, and a tolerance limit $\eta = 0.80$ are shown in Table 2.46, i.e., concentrations up to 6.25 are declared as non-toxic (further details are in Section 6.)

2.5.1.2 Proof of non-inferiority of poly-k estimates

The evaluation of tumor incidence in long-term rodent carcinogenicity studies without cause of death information can be performed by Cochran–Armitage-type [34] or Williams-type [299] trend tests for of proof of hazard. Using the multiple contrast approach, Dunnett-type confidence limits for poly-3 estimates were proposed [347]; see details in Section 3.5. This approach can be used for demonstrating non-inferiority without *a priori* defined tolerance limit by estimating the lower confidence limit. As a real data example, the incidences of skin fibromas on the carcinogenic potential of methyleugenol are used [314]. The time of death and the tumor status at the time of death were recorded for each animal; see the raw data in Table 3.10 in Section 3.5. Because increasing tumor rates are of toxicological interest, upper confidence limits are shown in Table 2.47 for claiming non-inferiority using the Add-1 Dunnett-type approach (see Section 2.1.5.3).

Table 2.47: Carcinogenicity Study on Methyleugenol

dose	0 mg/kg	37 mg/kg	75 mg/kg	150 mg/kg
No. tumors/No. animals	1/50	9/50	8/50	5/50
Crude tumor rates	0.02	0.18	0.16	0.10
Unadjusted upper confidence limits	-	0.18	0.25	0.28
Poly-3 adjusted n	41.4	40.3	38.7	32.7
Poly-3 adjusted rates	0.024	0.223	0.207	0.153
Poly-3 adjusted upper confidence limits	-	0.27	0.33	0.35

All poly-3 adjusted upper confidence limits are positive and rather large, therefore it is hard to conclude on non-inferiority and hence harmlessness on either dose group. Nowadays, the final tables for tumor evaluation in the NTP program reports already include the poly-3 adjusted rates, and we recommend to add the upper confidence limits and hints for their interpretation.

2.5.2 Two-sided hypotheses: Test on equivalence

Some endpoints in toxicology, such as body, litter, or organ weights, may show both increase or decrease. Therefore, the proof of safety is translated into a proof of equivalence. The new experimental treatments are declared to be safe/ equivalent to the control if they both do not undershoot a given fixed lower limit of the control and do not overshoot a given fixed upper limit of it, respectively. We additionally assume balancedness for the sample sizes of the experimental treatments, say $n_1 = \cdots = n_k$. The resulting component local tests are

$$H_{0i} : |\mu_i - \mu_0| \geq \delta \quad \text{vs.} \quad H_{1i} : |\mu_i - \mu_0| < \delta$$

with a relevant threshold $\delta > 0$. The global null hypothesis of the underlying union-intersection hypothesis (UIT) can be expressed as

$$H_0 = \bigcap_{i=1}^{k} H_{0i} = \bigcap_{i=1}^{k} \{H_{0i}^{(1)} \cup H_{0i}^{(2)}\}$$

with
$$H_{0i}^{(1)} : \mu_i - \mu_0 \le -\delta \quad \text{and} \quad H_{0i}^{(2)} : \mu_i - \mu_0 \ge \delta.$$

One can conclude equivalence for the ith treatment if

$$T_i(x_i, x_0) = \frac{|\bar{X}_i - \bar{X}_0| - \delta}{\hat{\sigma}\sqrt{\frac{1}{n_i} + \frac{1}{n_0}}} < -t_{k,1-\alpha}(\nu, \mathbf{R}).$$

with the lower $(1 - \alpha)$ quantile $t_{k,1-\alpha}(\nu, \mathbf{R})$ of an underlying k-variate t-distribution with correlation matrix $\mathbf{R} = (r_{ij})$ according to Bofinger and Bofinger [47] and [377].

The related confidence limits of the two-sided $(1 - \alpha)100\%$ SCI are given by

$$\hat{\delta}_i^l = \min\left(\bar{X}_i - \bar{X}_0 - t_{k,1-\alpha}(\nu, \mathbf{R}) S\sqrt{\frac{1}{n_i} + \frac{1}{n_0}}, 0\right),$$

$$\hat{\delta}_i^u = \max\left(\bar{X}_i - \bar{X}_0 + t_{k,1-\alpha}(\nu, \mathbf{R}) S\sqrt{\frac{1}{n_i} + \frac{1}{n_0}}, 0\right).$$

This approach is numerically available in the package ETC.

The body weights of a 90-day chronic toxicological study on rats with a control and three dose groups ([181]) will be evaluated here as an example.

```
> data("BW", package="ETC")
> BW$Dose <-as.factor(BW$Dose)
```

Although in the study decreasing body weights were observed (see the boxplots in Figure 2.34), an increased body weight would be a sign of toxicity too.

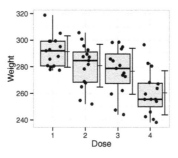

FIGURE 2.34: Boxplot for body weight data.

```
> library("ETC")
> comp <- etc.diff(formula=Weight~Dose,d ata=BW, margin.up=30,
+               method="Bofinger")
```

However, Bofinger's approach is limited to normal distributed endpoints, variance homogeneity, and balanced sample sizes in the treatment groups–rather restrictive assumptions for real toxicological studies. By taking into account the special structure of the correlation matrix, it becomes clear, that a Bonferroni-type alternative [151] does not lose much power even if all assumptions are fulfilled. It is much simpler and can be generalized for several situations [185]. We denote it here as the Bonferroni-TOST approach, because

Table 2.48: Simultaneous Bofinger-Type TOST Intervals for Body Weight Data

	2-1	3-1	4-1
lower	-22.88	-27.01	-43.28
upper	1.66	0.00	0.00

it is based on the two-one-sided-t-tests (TOST) and the multiplicity-adjustment according to Bonferroni. The Bonferroni-TOST approach can be formulated for any two-sample tests. As mentioned above, particularly relevant in toxicology are confidence intervals for ratio-to-control and where Bofinger's approach cannot be used: i) considering variance heterogeneity using Welch-t tests, ii) nonparametric intervals using Hodges–Lehmann intervals, iii) intervals for ratio-to-control in the case of variance homogeneity and heterogeneity. The above-mentioned body weight data is analyzed as ratio-to-control intervals for heterogeneous variances on the level $(1 - 2 * 0.05/3)$, where the number 2 comes from *two one-sided tests* and number 3 from *three comparisons versus control*.

```
> library("pairwiseCI")
> plot(pairwiseCI(Weight~Dose, data=BW, alternative = "two.sided",
+               conf.level = 1-2*0.05/3, method = "Param.ratio",
+               var.equal=FALSE, control=1), CIvert=FALSE,
+               H0line=c(0.8, 1, 1/0.8), H0lty=c(3,2,3))
```

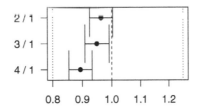

FIGURE 2.35: TOST intervals.

If we use the somewhat arbitrary $[0.8, 1.25]$ equivalence threshold from the bioequivalence framework, all doses will be declared as harmless.

3

Evaluation of long-term carcinogenicity assays

3.1 Principles

The purpose of a long-term carcinogenicity study is to evaluate the tumorigenic potency of a compound when it is administered to rodents for most of their life span [109, 270]. An FDA guideline describes study design and statistical analysis [14]. But, more in detail the US National Toxicology Program proposed a balanced design with a control and three dose groups with sample sizes of 50 animals for each sex and related statistical tests [9]. The primary objective is to identify a dose-dependent trend. Commonly the Cochran–Armitage test and its modifications are used. However, because of its limitations (see Section 2.1.6 for details), Williams-type tests (or just Dunnett-type tests for unrestricted comparisons against control) are used here. The primary endpoint in a carcinogenicity study is the number of tumors (more precisely the number of animals developing tumors). However, longer living animals develop tumors more likely than those dying earlier. Therefore the evaluation of crude tumor proportions could be biased, and thus both their mortality-adjusted analysis and the analysis of their survival as secondary endpoint are suggested. Commonly, the joint testing of age-adjusted tumor lethality (fatal tumors) and age-adjusted tumor prevalence (incidental tumors) is performed [300]. However, this classification based on the availability of the valid cause-of-death information for each individual tumor in each individual animal. In some studies this classification of a particular tumor into incidental, fatal, or mortality-independent is difficult or uncertain. As an alternative, the poly-k approach [34] was introduced where cause of death information is not necessary.

What is specific in the analysis of carcinogenicity assays?

1. The analysis of mortality, i.e., a Williams-type procedure for comparing survival functions

2. The analysis of crude tumor rates, i.e., a Williams-type procedure for proportions, particularly when the control rate tends to zero

3. The analysis of tumors taking the competing mortality into account using cause-of-death information or not

4. The analysis of rare tumors, particularly taking historical controls into account

5. The analysis of multiple tumors

6. The analysis of different-scaled responses, such as time-to-event and number of tumors

7. The combined analysis over sex

A debate exists whether to formulate one- or two-sided alternative hypotheses. Both allow directional decisions, however the first one at level α, the second one at level $\alpha/2$. Because the control of the false negative decision rate is important in toxicology, one-sided tests (and related confidence limits) should be used as long as the direction of harm can be unambiguously defined *a priori*. And without any doubt only potential increases in mortality or tumor rates are of interest in carcinogenicity studies.

Features:

- Test of crude tumor rates

- Williams-type trend test for survival functions, mortality-adjusted tumor rates with and without cause-of-death information

- Using historical tumor rates

3.2 Analysis of mortality

A naive analysis of the proportion of surviving animals summarized into a 2-by-k table can be performed by methods described in Section 2.1.5. But the comparison of the survival functions instead of crude proportions is more informative. The analysis of mortality is recommended by the US National Toxicology Program (NTP) [9], where p-values for a global trend test [369] and for pair-wise tests versus control [82] are described. In contrast, for the analysis of continuous variables they recommend the use of multiple comparison procedures, such as Dunnett [102] and Williams test [400, 401]. To overcome this contradiction, a Dunnett- and a Williams-type procedure for survival functions were proposed [158, 157] and used here in the examples.

3.2.1 Common NTP-style

Mortality data from the NTP study TR-120, a long-term *in vivo* bioassay of the carcinogenicity of piperonyl butoxide [13], are provided as an example. Survival was observed in three groups of female mice: a control group and two dose groups $[C, D_1, D_2]$, with 50 animals in each dose group and 20 animals in the control. The structure of the raw data is in a file format (see Table 3.1) with the variables: **chemical name, study no, Days DOSE_GROUP, Treatment, Event** (event=TRUE means animal died at that day), **REMOVAL- REASON** and **AnimalSex**. For the comparison of survival functions the factor **Treatment** and the variables **Days** and **Event** are relevant only.

```
> data("FMn", package="SiTuR")
```

Table 3.1: Raw Mortality Data of the TR-120 Bioassay

	Days	DOSE_GROUP	Treatment	Event	REMOVAL_REASON	AnimalSex
1	175	2500 PPM	D1	FALSE	Missing	FemaleMice
2	175	2500 PPM	D1	TRUE	Natural Death	FemaleMice
3	175	2500 PPM	D1	FALSE	Missing	FemaleMice
4	175	2500 PPM	D1	FALSE	Missing	FemaleMice
5	315	2500 PPM	D1	TRUE	Natural Death	FemaleMice
6	637	2500 PPM	D1	TRUE	Natural Death	FemaleMice

The Kaplan–Meier estimates are plotted in Figure 3.1, and we see dose-dependent survival functions. This plot can be suggested for a routine evaluation (together with their confidence bands).

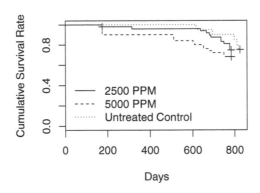

FIGURE 3.1: Kaplan–Meier plots for female mice in the TR120 bioassay.

As a next step, the mortality data are summarized into a 2-by-k table (see Table 3.2)

Table 3.2: 2-by-k Table of Mortality Data

	Control	D1	D2
surviving	15	38	34
dead	5	12	16
Total	20	50	50

Tarone's life table trend test [369] can be used within the library(coin) [194]. Here, a modification for a Williams-type permutation version is proposed. The contrast matrix for the two comparisons is defined by the function gW which is used in the argument xtrafo.

```
> library("coin")
> fm <- Surv(Days, Event) ~ Treatment
> Ch <- c(-1, 0,  1)
> Chm <- c(-1, .5,.5)
> gW <- function(x) {
+   x <- unlist(x)
+   cbind(High = Ch[x], All = Chm[x])
+ }
> itW <- independence_test(fm, data = FMn, xtrafo = gW,
+         distribution = approximate(B = 10000), alternative="greater")
> pvalTarone <-round(pvalue(itW, "single-step"), digits=3)
```

The one-sided p-value for a global increasing trend is 0.042 (i.e., for the comparison of high dose against control), where the p-value for the comparison of the control vs. the pooled medium and high dose is 0.069. Alternatively, two independent pairwise (control vs. dose) Cox proportional hazard models can be tested using the function coxph (see details in Section 3.2.2.

```
> library("survival")
> fm2500 <-droplevels(FMn[FMn$Treatment!="D2",])
> fm5000 <-droplevels(FMn[FMn$Treatment!="D1",])
> pval2500 <-round(summary(coxphFM <- coxph(Surv(Days, Event) ~ Treatment,
+                             data = fm2500))$waldtest[3], digits=3)
> pval5000 <-round(summary(coxphFM <- coxph(Surv(Days, Event) ~ Treatment,
+                             data = fm5000))$waldtest[3], digits=3)
```

The p-values for the comparison vs. the high dose is 0.0395 and vs. low dose is 0.097. Both approaches conclude a weak significant increase in mortality in the high dose only.

3.2.2   A Williams-type trend test for the comparison of survival functions

The Cox proportional hazards model $\lambda_i(t|i) = \lambda_0(t) \cdot \exp(\beta_i)$ describes the hazard rate for an animal in the ith group at time t, where $\lambda_0(t)$ is a baseline hazard rate assumed identical for all animals, and β_i is the effect of the ith treatment. A Williams-type test [400] can be formulated for $M = I - 1$ linear combinations of treatment effects $L_m = \sum_{i=1}^{I} c_{mi}\beta_i, \quad m = 1, ..., M.$. Approximate Wald-type lower simultaneous confidence intervals for the linear combinations L_m can be estimated [158]:

$$\sum_{i=1}^{I} c_{mi}\hat{\beta}_i - z_{M,\mathbf{R},1-\alpha}\sqrt{\sum_{i=1}^{I}\sum_{j=1}^{I} c_{mi}c_{mj}\hat{v}(\hat{\beta})_{ij}},$$

with $z_{M,\mathbf{R},1-\alpha}$ the equicoordinate $(1 - \alpha)$ quantile of the multivariate normal distribution with correlation matrix $\mathbf{R}$. Exponentiating the hazard ratio and the lower limits leads to simultaneous confidence intervals for multiple hazard ratios in the object FMCI:

```
> library("multcomp")
> coxphFM <- coxph(Surv(Days, Event) ~ Treatment, data = FMn)
> simCI.Williams.FM <- confint(glht(coxphFM,
+       linfct=mcp(Treatment="Williams"), alternative = "greater"))
> FMCI <- exp(simCI.Williams.FM$confint)
```

Table 3.3: Hazard Ratios and Their Lower Confidence Limits for Williams-Type Procedure on TR-120 Assuming a Cox Model

	Hazard ratio	Lower confidence limit
C 1	3.83	1.04
C 2	3.18	0.89

For the above NTP TR-120 study data, the hazard ratios and their lower confidence limits are given in Table 3.3, indicating a lightly significant monotone increasing mortality cause by the high-dose group (contrast C1). However, this tiny ratio of 1.039 indicates probably no relevant increase. Alternatively, a frailty Cox model can be used to model clustered survival data [375], e.g., to perform a joint analysis over both sexes or the two species mice and rats. This model accounts for possible heterogeneity between clusters by including a random cluster-specific intercept in the predictor of the Cox proportional hazards model; see further details in [157] (not shown here to keep the book simple).

3.3 Analysis of crude tumor rates

The analysis of crude tumor rates is quite common in both reports and publications. In a recent paper [38] the incidence of neoplasms in male and female B6C3F1 mice administered with 0, 0.0875, 0.175, 0.35, or 0.70 mmol acrylamide in the drinking water was evaluated (data taken from their Table 1). However, because of treatment-induced and/or tumor-induced mortality, conclusions from the analysis of crude tumors could be biased [34]. A further problem is the relatively small sample size, possibly aggravated by the mortality in the high-dose group. As an example, the two-year carcinogenicity study NTP558 [15] was selected.

```
> data("ntp558", package="SiTuR")
> ntp558$Treatment <- factor(ntp558$Treatment,
+                   levels=c("Control","Low","Medium","High"))
> nt558 <-table(ntp558$Tumor, ntp558$Treatment)
> rownames(nt558) <- c("Without Tumor", "With Tumor")
```

The summarized data are given in a 2-by-4 contingency table format in Table 3.4.

Table 3.4: 2-by-4 Table Summary of Crude Tumor Incidence of NTP588 Bioassay

	Control	Low	Medium	High
Without Tumor	50	46	46	44
With Tumor	0	4	4	6

Two approaches will be discussed in detail in the following Sections: i) a Williams-type trend test for proportions and ii) the analysis of tumor rates taking historical control data into account.

3.3.1 Analysis of crude tumor rates using a Williams-type test

The analysis of crude tumor rates is similar to the analysis of mortality proportions. For the NTP588 data, the Williams-type confidence limits and its point estimators of proportion difference to control are presented in Table 3.5 where small-sample-adjusted limits using the ADD1 approximation available in the library(MCPAN) was used (for further details see Section 2.1.5):

```
> library("MCPAN")
> lowerInt <-binomRDci(Tumor ~ Treatment, data=ntp558, type="Williams",
+          success="1", base=1, method="ADD1", alternative="greater")
```

All three contrasts reveal positive lower limits, with the contrast C3 (i.e., the global trend control vs. all pooled doses) showing the largest limit. A significantly increasing trend of tumor rates with a plateaus effect can be concluded.

Table 3.5: Williams-Type Lower Confidence Limits for Crude Tumor Rate

	Difference of proportion	Lower confidence limit
C 1	0.120	0.022
C 2	0.100	0.032
C 3	0.093	0.037

```
> library("MCPAN")
> lowerP <-binomRDtest(Tumor ~ Treatment, data=ntp558, type="Williams",
+                      success="1", base=1, method="ADD1",
+                      alternative="greater")$p.val.adj
```

Instead of confidence limits, one-sided multiplicity-adjusted p-values of 0.017, 0.004, 0.001 reveal a similar decision like the confidence limits, but in the scale of probabilities instead of rate differences.

3.3.2   Analysis of crude tumor rates using historical control data

A common practice in toxicology is to collect the historical control data of studies under similar conditions [153]. Particularly the historical tumor rates in carcinogenicity studies are used for the interpretation of rare tumors or unexpected in-/decreases in the concurrent control [108]. Starting from the pioneering paper [370] several proposals for including historical rates into a trend test on proportions are available. Recently, a related Williams-type procedure was proposed [215] providing simultaneous confidence intervals for small sample size designs. In the current assay, the number of tumors y_i in group i follows a binomial distribution $Bin(y_i|n_i, \pi_i)$. To incorporate the knowledge about the parameter π_i, a beta prior distribution $Beta(\pi_i|a_i, b_i)$ is used within an empirical Bayes approach. The corresponding posterior distribution is also a beta distribution with $Beta(\pi_i|a_i+y_i, b_i+n_i-y_i)$. Specifically for the control, the unknown parameters a_i and b_i are estimated from the beta-binomial model for the historical control data using the maximum likelihood method available in the package gamlss [321]. On the other hand, for the dose groups $i = 1, \dots, I$ a flat beta prior is assumed, which leads to parameter values of $a_i = 1$ and $b_i = 1$, the well-known ADD-2 approach [22]; see Table 3.6.

Table 3.6: Parameter Estimates for the Current Assay Resulting from a Beta Distribution with Informative (control group) and Uninformative (dose groups) Prior Distribution.

Estimate	Control group	Dose groups
proportion	$\hat{\pi}_0 = (\hat{a}_0 + y_0)/(\hat{a}_0 + \hat{b}_0 + n_0)$	$\hat{\pi}_i = (1 + y_i/(1 + 1 + n_i))$
sample size	$\hat{n}_0 = \hat{a}_0 + \hat{b}_0 + n_0$	$\hat{n}_i = 1 + 1 + n_i$

As a data example the crude proportion of alveolar/bronchial adenomas in mice after 102 weeks' exposure to pivalolactone and related historical rates from 23 bioassays are used here [358].

```
> data("HIST", package="SiTuR")
```

The boxplot in Figure 3.2 shows a descriptive summary of the historical tumor rates, superimposed with the tumor rates in the current study with doses 75 and 100 mg and the concurrent control (0) (points).

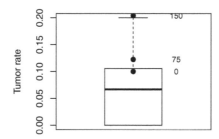

FIGURE 3.2: Boxplot for historical controls, superimposed by the proportion of the concurrent study.

Table 3.7: Williams-Type Lower Confidence Limits Using Historical Controls or Concurrent Control

	$DiffProp^{Concu}$	$lowerLimit^{Concu}$	$DiffProp^{Histo}$	$lowerLimit^{Histo}$
C 1	0.079	-0.084	0.131	0.021
C 2	0.040	-0.104	0.091	0.017

The Williams-type estimates and lower confidence limits of both approaches (concurrent control only/ with historical controls) are shown in Table 3.7. In this example the large concurrent control tumor rate of 2/20 is near to the 75% quantile of the historical rates. Therefore, the lower confidence limits are negative when considering the concurrent data only, i.e., claiming no increase in tumor rate. On the other hand, taking the historical controls into account reveals both positive confidence limits for the Williams-type contrasts C1 and C2. The difference between high dose and control is 0.021 and may indicate even a relevant increase.

This small example illustrates how important the use of the historical control information can be, especially from the perspective of the false negative rate, i.e., increasing the power to detect a difference. The relatively complex R-Code is not shown explicitly here to keep the book simple, but can be found in the knitr file according to [215].

3.4 Mortality-adjusted tumor rates with cause-of-death information

Approaches using cause-of-death information need the classification of each tumor into incidental, fatal, or observable. Tumors which are not responsible for death, but are observed at autopsy, e.g., caused by a different fatal tumor, are diagnosed as incidental. Tumors that kill the animal, are diagnosed as fatal. Observable tumors, such as skin tumors, are diagnosed as mortality independent and can be analyzed analogously to crude tumors (see above).

3.4.1 Analysis of incidental tumors

The idea is to partition the study period into a set of not too short time intervals (denoted as strata) together with the stratum for terminal sacrifices. The resulting stratified 2-by-k table is analyzed on dose-related trend where the stratified Cochran–Armitage test is commonly used. Notice, the test assumes a linear dose-response relationship which is not likely in carcinogenicity bioassays. An alternative is a Williams-type trend test on proportions [188]. Here a stratified permutation version is demonstrated by means of the R package `coin` [194]. As an example lung alveolar cell adenoma in male mice [1] is used.

```
> data("incidental", package="SiTuR")
> incidental$Dose <-factor(incidental$Treatment,
+                levels=c("Control", "Low", "Medium", "High")[c(1,2,3,4)])
```

The data were formally stratified into five time periods: the first year, up to 1.5 years, up to 91 weeks, the period of frequently occurring tumors between weeks 92 and 104, and finally the terminal sacrifice period; see the mosaic plot in Figure 3.3.

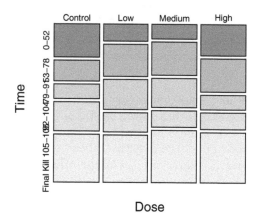

FIGURE 3.3: Mosaic plot of stratified lung alveolar cell adenoma.

This stratified 2-by-4 table was analyzed by a Williams-type trend test with the package `coin` using the contrast matrix in function `gWil`.

```
> library("coin")
> Ch <- c(-1, 0, 0, 1)
> Chm <- c(-1, 0, .5,.5)
> Chml <- c(-1, .33, .33, .33)
> gWill <- function(x) {
+ x <- unlist(x)
+ cbind(High = Ch[x], HighMed = Chm[x], All = Chml[x])
+ }
> williamInc<-pvalue(independence_test(Tumor ~ Dose | Time,
```

```
+              xtrafo = gWill, data = incidental, teststat = "maximum",
+              alternative = "less" ), method = "single-step")
```

Table 3.8: Williams-Type Multiplicity-Adjusted *p*-Values for an Incidental Tumor

	p-value
High	0.08
HighMed	0.13
All	0.31

The smallest one-sided adjusted *p*-value of 0.083 belongs to the comparison of the highest dose versus control and is larger than 0.05, i.e., no significant trend in the incidental lung alveolar cell adenoma can be concluded (see Table 3.8).

3.4.1.1   Further trend tests for stratified designs

Stratified designs occur frequently in toxicology, where a *stratum* represents a secondary, non-randomized factor, such as gender, species, or time-intervals for incidental tumors. The most common approach is the Mantel–Haenszel test (MH-test) [252]: per stratum a quadratic standardized test statistics is used and then summarized over the a strata. Either a χ^2 distribution with $df = a$ is used or a permutation approach [23] for such a global test. For a trend test a further problem occurs. Which contrasts should be used per stratum [238]? Assuming a stratum as a block factor, other possibilities exists, e.g., a fixed-effect model or a mixed-effect model. When using effect sizes such as odds ratios or risk differences the next problem is to find appropriate methods for small-sample confidence limits (see e.g., [217]). In Section 3.4.1 the permutative MH Williams-type trend test for the evaluation of incidental tumors is shown, whereas in Section 3.6.3 a similar Dunnett-type test with males and females as strata is used. Using the pre-neoplastic lesions in the olfactory epithelium from the carcinogenicity study on beta-picoline in B6C3F1 mice as an example [17], sex-specific strata are used for both fixed-effect and mixed-effect models to obtain Williams-type *p*-values.

```
> data("tr580", package="SiTuR")
```

In the fixed effect generalized linear model the factor Sex is used as a non-randomized block (without interaction between sex and dose) in the object fixM. The simultaneous Williams-type confidence intervals on the logit scale (left panel) show a significant increase. In the generalized mixed effect model Sex is used as a random factor (in the object fitSM) and the confidence limits are shown in the right panel, again with a significant increase.

```
> library("multcomp")
> par(mfrow=c(1,2))
> fixM <-glm(Tumor ~ Dose+ Sex, data = tr580,
+            family=binomial(link = "logit"))
> plot(glht(fixM, linfct = mcp(Dose = "Williams"),
+           alternative="greater"),  main="",
+           xlab=" ")
> library("lme4")
> fitSM <- glmer(Tumor~ Dose + (1|Sex), data=tr580,
```

```
+                family=binomial(link = "logit"))
> plot(glht(fitSM, linfct = mcp(Dose = "Williams"),
+           alternative="greater"), main="",
+           xlab="")

> stratP <-summary(glht(fitSM, linfct = mcp(Dose = "Williams"),
+                   alternative="greater"))
```

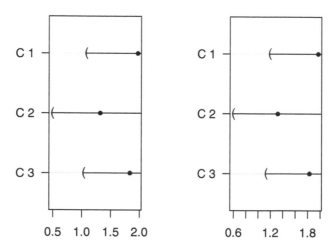

FIGURE 3.4: Williams-type *p*-values for fixed effect (left) or mixed effect (right) model in a stratified design.

Similar confidence limits are obtained for both approaches. And, the adjusted *p*-values of the mixed-effect model (in the object `stratP`) of 1.4×10^{-6}, 7.18×10^{-4}, 7×10^{-7} are also similar to those obtained with the permutation-based MH-trend test in Section 3.6.3. Comparison between these different combination styles and the different dose scores are needed before a certain approach can be suggested for the various stratified dose-response problems in toxicology.

In practice separate analysis of females and males is common; so the choice of sex as random seems rather arbitrary. Usually, long-term studies for both sexes as well as two species (usually rat and mice) are performed. Here, a joint analysis assuming the two random variables sex and species in the above style can be quite useful (see Section 3.6.3).

3.4.2   Analysis of fatal tumors

Since fatal tumors are responsible for observed mortality, the log-rank test can be used for their analysis [250], particularly its permutative version for small sample sizes. As an example the NTP three-year carcinogenicity study TR 558 on tetrachloroazobenzene in Sprague–Dawley rats was used, from which the data of liver cholangiocarcinoma in male rats were selected [15].

```
> data("ntp558", package="SiTuR")
> ntp558$Treatment <- factor(ntp558$Treatment,
```

```
+                          levels=c("Control","Low","Medium","High"))
> nt558 <-table(ntp558$Tumor, ntp558$Treatment)
> rownames(nt558) <- c("Without Tumor", "With Tumor")
```

Th related Kaplan–Meier estimators are shown in Figure 3.5.

```
> library("survival")
> plot(survfit(Surv(Weeks, Censoring) ~ Treatment, data = ntp558),
+       main = "Weeks to first liver cholangiocarcinoma
+       in male rats NTP-558", cex.main=0.7,
+       lty = 1:3, xlab="Weeks", ylab="Cumulative Tumor-free Rate")
> legend("bottomleft", lty = 1:3, levels(ntp558$Treatment), bty = "n")
```

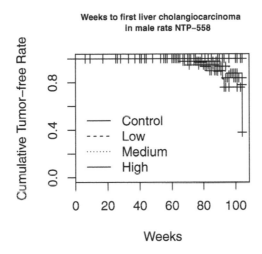

FIGURE 3.5: Kaplan-Meier estimator for fatal liver cholangiocarcinoma.

For a Dunnett-type version of the permutation log-rank test using the correlation matrix in function DUN, all three one-sided p-values are less than 0.05 and therefore an increase in the liver cholangiocarcinoma occurs in the low, medium, and high dose (see Table 3.9).

```
> library("coin")
> Cm <- c(-1, 0, 0, 1)
> Cl <- c(-1, 0, 1, 0)
> Ch <- c(-1, 1, 0, 0)
> DUN <- function(x) {
+ x <- unlist(x)
+ cbind(CvsLow = Cl[x], CvsMed = Cm[x], CvsHigh = Ch[x])
+ }
> dunnettFAT<- pvalue(independence_test(Surv(Weeks, Censoring)~Treatment,
+                   data =ntp558, xtrafo =DUN, teststat = "maximum",
+                   alternative="greater",
+                   distribution = approximate(B = 10000)),
+                   method = "single-step")
```

Table 3.9: Dunnett-Type One-sided Adjusted p-Values for Fatal Tumor Evaluation

	p-value
CvsLow	1.0000
CvsMed	1.0000
CvsHigh	1.0000

3.5   Mortality-adjusted tumor rates without cause-of-death information

The poly-k trend test was developed as an alternative if cause-of-death information is not available or uncertain [34, 41]. This test is a modification of the Cochran–Armitage test ([31], i.e., a linear trend test of mortality-adjusted tumor rates. Simulation studies showed that the poly-k test performed well under many conditions and is robust to different tumor lethality patterns [266]. Appealing is its simplicity: the analysis of crude proportions is replaced by poly-k adjusted proportions. Therefore, the poly-k test and its bootstrap-based version [267] is the standard approach for evaluating long-term carcinogenicity studies of the US National Toxicology Program (NTP). Since the Cochran–Armitage test has the disadvantage of testing almost linear trends, related approximate multiple contrast tests of the Dunnett- and Williams-type and particularly their simultaneous confidence intervals on the poly-3 adjusted tumor rates were proposed [347] as an alternative. The basic idea is to account for censoring due to treatment-specific mortality by individual weights $w_{ij} = (t_{ij}/t_{max})^k$ reflecting individual mortality pattern (t_{ij} is time of death of animal j in treatment i). $k = 3$ seems to be a good choice. These weights result in adjusted sample sizes $n_i^* = \sum_{j=1}^{n_i} w_{ij}$ (which are used instead of the randomized number of animals n_i). Therefore adjusted proportions $p_i^* = y_i/n_i^*$ are used instead of the crude tumor proportions $p_i = y_i/n_i$ in Dunnett/Williams-type procedures. As an example the NTP study on the carcinogenic potential of methyleugenol for the incidence of skin fibromas is used [314].

```
> data("methyl", package="MCPAN")
```

Table 3.10 contains in the first two rows the unadjusted crude tumor rates and in rows 3 - 4 the mortality-adjusted rates. In the dose groups the adjusted rates p_i^* are substantially increased, reflecting a competing mortality.

Table 3.10: Crude and Poly-3-Adjusted Tumor Rates in the Methyleugenol Study

dose	0 mg/kg	37 mg/kg	75 mg/kg	150 mg/kg
Crude Rate	1/50	9/50	8/50	5/50
Crude Percent	2.0%	18.0%	16.0%	10.0%
Poly-3 adjusted Rate	1/41.4	9/40.3	8/38.7	5/32.7
Poly-3 adjusted Percent	2.4%	33.3%	30.7%	15.3%

We consider one-sided hypotheses and therefore one-sided Dunnett-type tests and one-sided confidence limits, because only increasing tumor rates are of interest.

```
> library("MCPAN")
> plot(poly3ci(time=methyl$death, status=methyl$tumour,
+            f=methyl$group, type = "Dunnett", method = "ADD1",
+            alternative="greater"), lines=0)
```

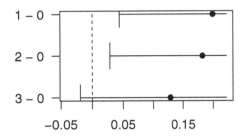

FIGURE 3.6: Lower Dunnett-type confidence limits for poly-3 adjusted tumor rates.

According to Section 2.1.5.3 the confidence intervals are based on the ADD-1 adjustment using $p_i^* = (y_i + 0.5) / (n_i^* + 1)$. The confidence limits plot in Figure 3.6 indicates an increase of the mortality-adjusted tumor rates in the low (1) and medium dose (2), but not in the high dose (3).

In a recent publication [222] a clear statement to recommend the poly-3 tests is missing. However, when comparing the simplicity and the possible loss of efficiency of the poly-3 tests with respect to the almost always more complex analysis of incidental/fatal tumors, a clear recommendation as routine method follows from my perspective.

3.6 More complex analyzes

3.6.1 Multiple tumors

Multiple tumors occur commonly: i) in several organs or systems, ii) as specific classifications (i.e., adenomas, carcinoma, metastasizing carcinomas), iii) in different entities within an organ-specific carcinoma (e.g., hepatocellular carcinoma, hepatocholangiocarcinoma), and iv) in paired organs (e.g., multiple locations in mammary glands). Commonly, all these many tumors are analyzed independently, i.e., many univariate tests at level α are used. According to the large number of multiple tumors, even > 100 in some bioassays, the false positive decision rate increases and a multiplicity adjustment within the proof of hazard was recommended [59]. This dimension of multiplicity increases, furthermore, when independent two-sample tests for the comparison of dose groups against the control are performed; see e.g., the 24 individual permutative Fisher tests for the 6 tumors and 4 doses in the 80-week carcinogenesis bioassay with female mice in the SAS program multtest [392]. Here, the contradiction between the control of the familywise error rate (global test to adjust against multiple tumors and multiple comparisons vs. control) and control of the comparisonwise error rate (each tumor and each comparison vs. control is tested independently at level α) gapes significantly. In the toxicological interpretation it should be noted that the first approach is over-conservative, whereas the second is over-liberal. The challenge for a global test is the modeling of the correlation between these individual tumors, i.e., first which tumors occur in the same animal simultaneously and second which correlation between the treatment comparisons occurs. A maximum test can be used to adjust against the p tumors. Consequently, a max-max-test for adjustment against p tumors *and* k group comparisons simultaneously is needed. The challenge is to take this complex correlation matrix into account. This can be done by i) a permutation approach [192, 393], ii) the explicit formulation of the correlation matrix to use a central pk-variate normal distribution [145], or iii) marginal model approach [307]. The first and third approaches will be demonstrated by means of an example here (the second approach is only available for normal distributed endpoints up to now). As an example for multiple tumors data from the NTP bioassay on methyleugenol (No. TR491) in female mice with tumors from 89 tumor sites were selected [314]. The dataset contains the tumor counts together with the dose group (0, 37, 75, and 150 mg/kg) and the time of death.

```
> data("miceF", package="SiTuR")
```

To keep the problem tractable for demonstration purposes, adenomas and carcinomas of the liver were selected (abbreviated with *t19: carcinoma, metastatic ureter carcinoma, t20: metastatic mesentery fibrosarcoma, t21: metastatic skin fibrosarcoma, t22: hemangioma, t23: metastatic spleen hemangiosarcoma, t24: hepatoblastoma, t25: multiple hepatoblastoma, t26: hepatocellular adenoma, t27: multiple hepatocellular adenoma, t28: hepatocellular carcinoma, t29: multiple hepatocellular carcinoma, t30: hepatocholangiocarcinoma, t31: histiocytic sarcoma, t32: malignant mast cell tumor, t33: uncertain osteosarcoma, t34: malignant plasma cell tumor and t35: malignant schwannoma*).

To highlight the correlation between the tumors, the raw data are given in Table 3.11 where each single row represents an animal (and the factor **group** is abbreviated with **Gr**).

Table 3.11: Raw Multiple Tumor Data

t19	t20	t21	t22	t23	t24	t25	t26	t27	t28	t29	t30	t31	t32	t33	t34	t35	Gr
0	0	0	0	0	0	0	0	0	0	0	0	0	0	0	0	0	0
0	0	0	0	0	0	0	0	0	0	0	0	0	0	0	0	0	0
0	0	0	0	0	0	0	0	0	0	0	0	0	0	0	0	0	0
0	0	0	0	0	0	0	0	0	0	0	0	0	0	0	0	0	0
0	0	0	0	0	0	0	0	0	0	0	0	0	0	0	0	0	0
0	0	0	0	0	0	0	0	0	0	0	0	0	0	0	0	0	0
0	0	0	0	0	0	0	0	0	0	0	0	0	0	0	0	0	0
0	0	0	0	0	0	0	0	0	0	0	0	0	0	0	0	0	0
0	0	0	0	0	0	0	0	1	0	0	0	0	0	0	0	0	0
0	0	0	0	0	0	0	0	0	1	0	0	0	0	0	0	0	0
...	...	...	...	...	...	...	...	...	...	...	...	...	...	...	...	...	...
0	0	0	0	0	0	0	0	0	0	1	0	0	0	0	0	0	3
0	0	0	0	0	0	0	1	0	0	1	0	0	0	0	0	0	3
0	0	0	0	0	0	1	0	0	1	0	0	0	0	0	0	0	3
0	0	0	0	0	1	0	0	0	0	1	0	0	0	0	0	0	3
0	0	0	0	0	0	0	1	0	0	1	0	0	0	0	0	0	3
0	0	0	0	0	1	0	0	1	0	1	0	0	0	0	0	0	3
0	0	0	0	0	1	0	0	1	0	1	0	0	0	0	0	0	3
0	0	0	0	0	1	0	0	1	1	0	0	0	0	0	0	0	3
0	0	0	0	0	0	1	0	0	0	1	0	0	0	0	0	0	3

The tumor incidences are visualized in the mosaic plot in Figure 3.7. Tumor sites t24, t25, t27, and t29 appear to have a treatment or even a trend effect, the others show only sporadic tumors. Notice, the tumor sites t25 and t29 reveal only zeros in the control.

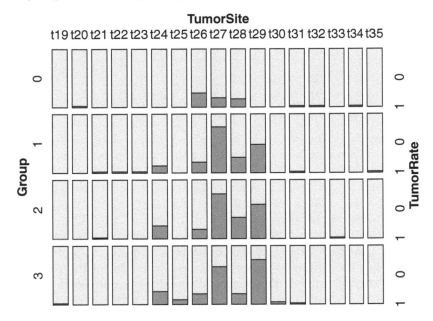

FIGURE 3.7: Mosaic plot for multiple liver tumors.

Following the pioneering paper [59] permutation tests are commonly used. As an alternative to pairwise Fisher tests [392] the rather conservative Dunnett-type approach for multiple binary endpoints within the framework of conditional inference is used by means of the package coin [194].

```
> library("coin")
> aa <- c(0,0,0,1)
> dd <- c(0,0,1,0)
> rr <- c(0,1,0,0)
> g <- function(x) {
+     x <- unlist(x)
+     cbind( CD1 = rr[x], CD2 = dd[x],CD3 = aa[x])
+ }
> it <- independence_test(t19+t20+t21+t22+t23+t24+t25+
+     t26+t27+t28+t29+t30+t31+t32+t33+t34+t35
+      ~ Group, data = miceL,  xtrafo = g, alternative = "greater")
> pvalM <- matrix(round(pvalue(it, method = "single-step"), 4), nr = 3)
```

Table 3.12: *p*-Values for Dunnett-Type Tests for Multiple Tumors—I

	t19	t20	t21	t22	t23	t24	t25	t26	t27
Low vs. C	1.00	1.00	1.00	0.89	0.89	1.00	1.00	1.00	0.03
Mid vs. C	1.00	1.00	1.00	1.00	1.00	0.80	1.00	1.00	0.09
High vs. C	0.89	1.00	1.00	1.00	1.00	0.80	0.01	1.00	1.00

The multiplicity-adjusted *p*-values (adjusted both against 17 tumor sites and 3 treatment comparisons!) are given in Table 3.12, whereas t25 (in the high dose), t27 (in the low dose), and t29 (in the high dose) reveal a significantly increasing effect.

Table 3.13: *p*-Values for Dunnett-Type Tests for Multiple Tumors—II

	t28	t29	t30	t31	t32	t33	t34	t35
Low vs. C	1.00	1.00	1.00	1.00	1.00	1.00	1.00	0.89
Mid vs. C	0.34	0.65	1.00	1.00	1.00	0.89	1.00	1.00
High vs. C	1.00	0.00	0.30	1.00	1.00	1.00	1.00	1.00

Recently, several papers for the evaluation of correlated binary data were published: order restricted tests [88, 87] or simultaneous confidence intervals for two-sample design [218]. However, either no software is available or a personalized code only. An alternative is simultaneous inference (i.e., adjusted *p*-values and/or confidence intervals) based on tumor-specific generalized linear models (using binomial link function) and the use of their parameter estimates to derive the joint asymptotic distribution [307]. This approach allows the extension to several groups and the use of many-to-one comparisons (i.e., Dunnett-type approach) or order restricted tests (i.e., Williams-type approach). A problem of unstable model fits arises when the parameter estimates is near to border of the parameter space, e.g., when all or nearly all animals in the control reveal no tumor, particularly for small sample size designs. Several solutions can be used; here we use the simple ADD-2 approach [346] on a table data level. By means of the `mmm` function in the R package `multcomp` the example data can be analyzed accordingly. The object `multT` contains the simultaneous estimates based on the individual generalized linear model estimates for each tumor in the objects `glm19,...,glm35`:

```
> library("multcomp")
> glm19 <- glm(cbind(Successes + 1, 52 - (Successes+1)) ~ Group,
+             subset(miceN, Site=="t19"), family=binomial())
> glm20 <- glm(cbind(Successes + 1, 52 - (Successes+1)) ~ Group,
+             subset(miceN, Site=="t20"), family=binomial())
> glm21 <- glm(cbind(Successes + 1, 52 - (Successes+1)) ~ Group,
+             subset(miceN, Site=="t21"), family=binomial())
> glm22 <- glm(cbind(Successes + 1, 52 - (Successes+1)) ~ Group,
+             subset(miceN, Site=="t22"), family=binomial())
> glm23 <- glm(cbind(Successes + 1, 52 - (Successes+1)) ~ Group,
+             subset(miceN, Site=="t23"), family=binomial())
> glm24 <- glm(cbind(Successes + 1, 52 - (Successes+1)) ~ Group,
+             subset(miceN, Site=="t24"), family=binomial())
> glm25 <- glm(cbind(Successes + 1, 52 - (Successes+1)) ~ Group,
+             subset(miceN, Site=="t25"), family=binomial())
> glm26 <- glm(cbind(Successes + 1, 52 - (Successes+1)) ~ Group,
+             subset(miceN, Site=="t26"), family=binomial())
> glm27 <- glm(cbind(Successes + 1, 52 - (Successes+1)) ~ Group,
+             subset(miceN, Site=="t27"), family=binomial())
> glm28 <- glm(cbind(Successes + 1, 52 - (Successes+1)) ~ Group,
+             subset(miceN, Site=="t28"), family=binomial())
> glm29 <- glm(cbind(Successes + 1, 52 - (Successes+1)) ~ Group,
+             subset(miceN, Site=="t29"), family=binomial())
> glm30 <- glm(cbind(Successes + 1, 52 - (Successes+1)) ~ Group,
+             subset(miceN, Site=="t30"), family=binomial())
> glm31 <- glm(cbind(Successes + 1, 52 - (Successes+1)) ~ Group,
+             subset(miceN, Site=="t31"), family=binomial())
> glm32 <- glm(cbind(Successes + 1, 52- (Successes+1)) ~ Group,
```

```
+                subset(miceN, Site=="t32"), family=binomial())
> glm33 <- glm(cbind(Successes + 1, 52 - (Successes+1)) ~ Group,
+                subset(miceN, Site=="t33"), family=binomial())
> glm34 <- glm(cbind(Successes + 1, 52 - (Successes+1)) ~ Group,
+                subset(miceN, Site=="t34"), family=binomial())
> glm35 <- glm(cbind(Successes + 1, 52 - (Successes+1)) ~ Group,
+                subset(miceN, Site=="t35"), family=binomial())
> multT <-glht(mmm(T19=glm19,T20=glm20,T21=glm21,T22=glm22,T23=glm23,
+                   T24=glm24,T25=glm25,T26=glm26,T27=glm27,T28=glm28,
+                   T29=glm29,T30=glm30,T31=glm31,T32=glm32,T33=glm33,
+                   T34=glm34,T35=glm35),
+                 mlf(mcp(Group ="Dunnett")), alternative="greater")
```

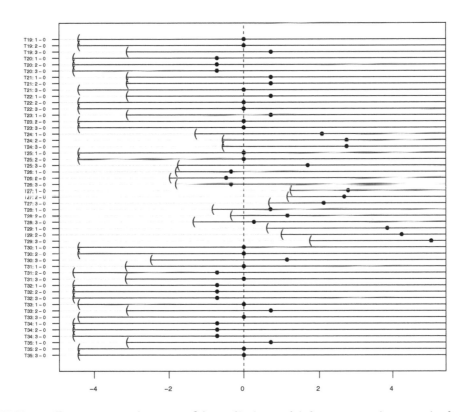

FIGURE 3.8: Dunnett-type lower confidence limits multiple tumors using marginal models.

Figure 3.8 contains the lower simultaneous confidence limits, where tumors t24, t27, and t29 reveal significant increasing tumor rates (alternatively the multiplicity-adjusted p-values can be estimated via `fortify(summary(multT))[, c(1,6)]`).

Summarizing, the joint analysis of multiple tumors is still delicate and cannot be recommended in the routine work. If needed, the transparent and simple Bonferroni-adjustment should be used because its power is not substantially reduced with respect to permutation tests [218] (not shown here).

3.6.2   Multivariate response

The joint analysis of three response endpoints: i) survival time, ii) time to first tumor, and iii) total number of tumors of animals in different treatment groups was demonstrated by the R package coin [193] using the photococarcinogenicity data [264] in the example part of this package. The difference between multiple tumors and multivariate response is: i) multiple endpoints are on the same scale (i.e., commonly proportions), but ii) different-scaled endpoints are analyzed in the multivariate setup. As an example, data of female mice are used, which were exposed to different levels of ultraviolet radiation (group A with topical vehicle and 600 units, group B 600 units only, and group C 1200 units only). Figure 3.9 demonstrates the treatment effects for all three response endpoints [193, 192, 194]. The three above-mentioned primary endpoints are available.

```
> data("photocar", package="coin")
```

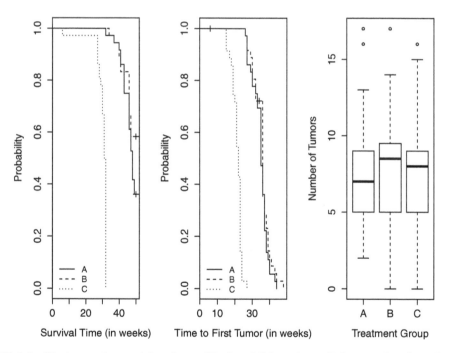

FIGURE 3.9: Photocarcinogenicity data: Kaplan-Meier plots of time to death and time to first tumor as well as boxplots of the total number of tumors.

First, a global test for the null hypothesis of the independence between the treatment levels and *all* three response variables is used. A max-type test based on the standardized multivariate linear statistic and an approximation of the conditional distribution utilizing the asymptotic distribution simply reads:

```
> library("coin")
> aa <- c(0,0,1)
> dd <- c(0,1,0)
> gP <- function(x) {
+     x <- unlist(x)
```

```
+       cbind(Cvs.D2 = aa[x], Cvs.D1 = dd[x])
+ }
> it_ph <- independence_test(Surv(time, event) +
+           Surv(dmin, tumor) + ntumor ~ group,
+           xtrafo = gP, data = photocar)
```

Here, the influence function consists of a sum of the log-rank scores of the survival time, the time to first tumor, and the number of tumors.

Table 3.14: Multiplicity-Adjusted p-Values of Photocarcinogencity Example

	Survival time	Time to first tumor	No. of tumors
Cvs.D2	0.000000	0.000000	0.997100
Cvs.D1	0.000000	0.000200	1.000000

In Table 3.14 we can see the rejection of the global null hypothesis is due to the group differences in both survival time and time to first tumor whereas no treatment effect on the total number of tumors can be observed.

3.6.3   The combined analysis over sex

The common bioassays with both sexes and two species (mice, rats) are analyzed independently. However, sometimes a joint analysis is more appropriate. As an example the incidences of the non-neoplastic lesion metaplasia of olfactory epithelium in both male and female mice in the NTP TR-580 for beta-picoline is used [17].

```
> data("tr580", package="SiTuR")
```

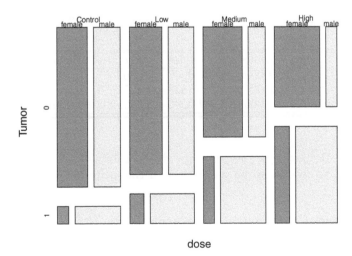

FIGURE 3.10: Incidence of metaplasia of olfactory epithelium in both male and female mice in the TR-580 bioassay.

The structure of the data is visualized in the mosaic plot in Figure 3.10. The secondary factor can be seen as a block factor, and therefore for this stratified design the Cochran–Mantel–Haenszel test can be used. Particularly simple is the conditional inference with the package coin, where the permutations are within each stratum to compute stratum-specific expectation and covariance which are finally aggregated over all strata [192, 194, 193]. The example is analyzed for: i) the pooled data in object dP580(not recommended), ii) sex-separated in the objects dm580, fm580, and iii) stratified in the object startif:

```
> library("coin")
> add <- c(0, 0, 0, 1)
> dom <- c(0, 0, 1, 0)
> rec <- c(0, 1, 0, 0)
> g <- function(x) {
+   x <- unlist(x)
+   cbind(CvsHigh = add[x], CvsMed = dom[x], CvsLow = rec[x])
+ }
> stratif <- independence_test(Tumor ~ dose | Sex, data = tr580,
+                              xtrafo = g, alternative = "greater")
> pstrat <-pvalue(stratif, method = "single-step")
> m580 <-tr580[tr580$Sex=="male", ]
> f580 <-tr580[tr580$Sex=="female", ]
> dm580 <- independence_test(Tumor ~ dose, data = m580,
+                            xtrafo = g, alternative = "greater")
> df580 <- independence_test(Tumor ~ dose , data = f580,
+                            xtrafo = g, alternative = "greater")
> pm <-pvalue(dm580, method = "single-step")
> pf <-pvalue(df580, method = "single-step")
> dP580 <- independence_test(Tumor ~ dose , data = tr580,
+                            xtrafo = g, alternative = "greater")
> pp <-pvalue(dP580, method = "single-step")
```

Table 3.15: Dunnett-Type p-Values for Pooled, Sex-Specific and Stratified Analysis

	Pooled	Males	Females	Stratified
CvsHigh	0.0000000	0.0000000	0.0007567	0.0000000
CvsMed	0.0656258	0.0173833	0.9272024	0.0469957
CvsLow	1.0000000	1.0000000	0.9999996	1.0000000

The related adjusted Dunnett-type p-values are given in Table 3.15, where the advantage of stratified tests can be seen from the comparison of the medium dose against control.

3.6.4   Time-to-event data with litter structure

Litter-matched time-to-response carcinogenicity data represents a rather specific structure of a teratogenicity study (available in the dataset km [251]; see the raw data in Table 3.16). In this two-sample design (factor treatment with level 0 ...control or 1... treated) several values are available: i) the time until an animal developed a tumor (time), ii) the status whether with or without tumor (tumor), and iii) the censoring status (censored) (here rather specific because only with the final sacrifice period). (Notice, Litter| is a factor.)

```
> data("km", package="SiTuR")
> km$Treatment <- as.factor(km$treatment)
> km$Litter <- as.factor(km$litter)
```

Table 3.16: Litter-Matched Time-to-Response Raw Data

time	tumor	treatment	litter	censored	Treatment	Litter
34	1	1	30	0	1	30
39	1	1	13	0	1	13
40	1	0	23	0	0	23
45	0	0	13	0	0	13
45	1	1	35	0	1	35
...	...	...	...	...		
104	0	1	21	1	1	21
104	0	1	22	1	1	22
104	0	1	23	1	1	23
104	0	1	25	1	1	25
104	0	1	28	1	1	28
104	0	1	37	1	1	37
104	0	1	38	1	1	38
104	0	1	44	1	l	44
104	0	1	50	1	1	50

Possible approaches for these clustered time-to-event data are Dunnett-type tests based on a frailty Cox model [157]:

```
> library("survival")
> cpl <- coxph(Surv(time, !censored)~ Treatment + frailty(Litter), data=km)
> library("multcomp")
> hrcpl <- glht(cpl, mcp(Treatment="Dunnett"),alternative = "greater")
> frailt <-exp(confint(hrcpl)$confint)
```

or a mixed effect Cox-model where `litter` is used as a random factor:

```
> library("coxme")
> svcme <- coxme(Surv(time, !censored) ~ Treatment + (1|litter), data = km)
> CIscme <- confint(glht(svcme, linfct=mcp(Treatment="Dunnett"),
+                        alternative = "greater"))
> come <-exp(CIscme$confint)
```

The effect size is the hazard rate of 1.39 where the lower confidence limit for the frailty model is 0.943 (in the object `frailt`) which is similar to that of the random-effects Cox model 0.947 (in the object `come`).

4

Evaluation of mutagenicity assays

4.1 What is specific in the analysis of mutagenicity assays?

It is no coincidence that the most cited work in the last few years refers to the Comet assay [247]. Yes, the various *in vitro* and *in vivo* mutagenicity bioassays make substantial demands on the statistical method. Selected issues are formulated in the following 12 special features:

1. The concentrations used particularly in *in vitro* assays are somewhat arbitrary in relation to the exposure to humans. Therefore, a tendency to overdosing exists to avoid false negative results. A specific dose-response problem may occur: downturn effects at high(er) concentrations. Trend tests assuming strict order restriction may be seriously biased and therefore a downturn-protected trend test or a one-sided comparison versus control without order restriction (Dunnett-type procedure) is proposed. As an example, Ames assay data are analyzed accordingly; see Section 4.2.

2. Most endpoints are counts, such as number of revertants or number of micronuclei. Therefore appropriate procedures for the analysis of counts per experimental unit (i.e., animal or plate) are needed. Among others, four approaches are described here: i) generalized linear mixed model for Poisson variables (see Section 4.6), ii) generalized linear model for overdispersed Poisson variables (see Section 4.6), iii) nonparametric approach allowing ties (see Section 4.3) and iv) data-transformation for the approximate use of parametric approaches (see Section 4.7).

3. Very small sample sizes are commonly used in both *in vitro* and *in vivo* assays, such as triplicate plates in the Ames assay or 5 mice in the micronucleus assay. This rather critical limitation from a statistical perspective is discussed for the proposed statistical approaches. As an example an *in vivo* micronucleus assay is evaluated; see Section 4.3.

4. Zero or near-to-zero counts or proportions in the control occur in some assays, particularly for pathological response endpoints, such as number of tumors, foci, or micronuclei. A simple transformation procedure will be discussed and demonstrated for the evaluation of HET-MN assay (see Section 4.7). Alternatively, a profile likelihood approach is used to analyze the cell transformation assay data (see Section 4.8.1).

5. Instead of evaluating just counts, sometimes the number at risk should be considered and therefore procedures for proportions are discussed as well. Commonly, a trend test for proportions is of primary interest. As an example, the number of morphologically transformed colonies per total number of scored colonies in SHE assay are evaluated; see Section 4.4. Moreover, modifications of the common-used CA-trend test (see Section 4.4.1), a global test followed by pairwise tests (see Section 4.4.2) as well as Dunnett/Williams-type procedures for proportions (see Section 4.4.3) are discussed.

6. Instead of analyzing 2-by-k table data, proportions may vary between animals in *in vivo* studies, such as the micronucleus assays. Therefore, procedures taking the overdispersion into account are discussed (see Section 4.5).

7. In some assays biological relevance is characterized by a k-fold rule, i.e., a change threshold. Therefore, procedures for ratio-to-control are proposed and demonstrated using the LLNA assay as an example; see Section 4.9.

8. The use of historical control data can be helpful. A particular approach for the analysis of micronuclei counts is described in Section 4.10.

9. Current assay sensitivity is sometimes proofed by comparing the positive control against the negative control. As an example an *in vivo* micronucleus assay is used; see Section 4.11.

10. When analyzing the Comet assay data, e.g., focusing on the endpoint tail moment, the question arises why 100 cells are analyzed and not just one or two. One answer is that the pathological effect of extreme enlargement occurs only in some cells whereas the majority of the cells remain unaffected. Therefore the use of common tests on mean differences may be inappropriate. Alternatively we can assume a mixing distribution of many non-responders and some responders. This complex approach is demonstrated in Section 4.12.

11. A relevant issue is the distinction between a randomized unit, such as an animal, and technical (non-randomized) replicates: cells within slides/ slides within samples/ samples within organs and organs within the randomized animal in the Comet assay. A possible approach is demonstrated in Section 4.12.

12. In the *in vitro* micronuclei assay one strategy is to compare cell distributions instead of several independent counts. Therefore in Section 4.13 simultaneous inference for multinomial distributions is discussed.

Features:

- Evaluation of proportions or counts with or without extra-binomial variability
- Evaluation of near-to-zero counts
- Assuming a mixing distribution of responders and non-responders
- Analyzing cell distribution by inference on multinomials
- Taking either historical controls or the positive control into account

---

4.2 Evaluation of the Ames assay as an example for dose–response shapes with possible downturn effects

According to Paracelsus law *Dosis sola venenum facit* [49] is the dose-response analysis a central issue in toxicology. Monotonic shapes are commonly assumed, sometimes even the rather specific case of a linear curve using logarithmic dose metameters [386]. In contrast, non-monotonic shapes are not too rare, e.g., in studies with endocrine disruptors [382, 350] or for the neurotoxicity of methylmercury [394]. Non-monotonicity at low doses (hormesis) or high doses (downturn effect) may occur. In the following the evaluation of downturn effects will be discussed only. Concentrations used in *in-vitro* assay are not necessarily related to human target concentrations and therefore a tendency for over-dosing exists in mutagenicity assays to avoid false negative decisions. A downturn effect at high(er) concentrations may therefore occur. An impressive example is the dataset of the Ames assay with TA98 [255] with a clear downturn effect at doses higher than $100\mu g$; see Figure 4.1. A simple recommendation for testing such dose-response curves is to use the two-sided Dunnett procedure which detects changes to control for all dose groups in any direction. However, a significantly increasing dose-related trend is used as causation criterion, e.g., for the *in vitro* micronucleus assay [290]. Therefore the detection of a trend up to a peak point dose is needed. The use of a global trend test with strict monotone alternative may be seriously biased (although the Williams-type approach is to some extent robust due to its pooling-contrasts property) and a trend test up to the visually observed peak point dose cannot control the familywise error rate (FWER). Therefore a multiple contrast test for all monotone alternatives up to all possible peak point doses was proposed [54]. Because the k-fold rule is used for the Ames-assay, the ratio-to-control comparison version is used here [97] as an example. The nominator contrast matrix is shown in Table 4.1 (whereas in the denominator matrix in the first row are 1's for ratio-to-control comparisons).

```
> data("salmonella", package="aod")
> salmonella$Dose <-as.factor(salmonella$dose)
```

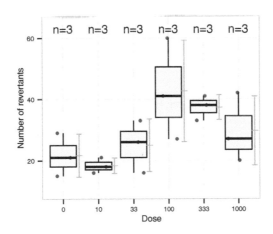

FIGURE 4.1: Boxplots of TA98 Ames assay.

The basic idea is to construct a multiple contrast test for Williams-type contrasts for all $k, (k-1), ..., 1$ possible peak point doses $(PPD_{1000}, PPD_{333}, PPD_{100}, PPD_{33}, PPD_{10})$; see Table 4.1.

The contrasts C1 to C5 belong to a global Williams-type test (assuming the peak point dose is $D_5 = 1000$), the contrasts C6-C9 to a partial Williams-type test (assuming the peak point dose is $D_4 = 333$), etc. Figure 4.2 shows the one-sided lower limits for these 15 comparisons from C1 (PPD1000 1000/0) up to C15 (PPD10, 10/0).

Table 4.1: Nominator Contrast Matrix for Downturn Protected Williams-Type Test

	0	10	33	100	333	1000
C1:PPD1000|1000-0	0.00	0.00	0.00	0.00	0.00	1.00
C2:PPD1000|(1000+333)/2-0(C2)	0.00	0.00	0.00	0.00	0.50	0.50
C3:PPD1000|(1000+333+100)3-0	0.00	0.00	0.00	0.33	0.33	0.33
C4:PPD1000|(1000+333+100+33)/4-0	0.00	0.00	0.25	0.25	0.25	0.25
C5:PPD1000|(1000+333+100+33+10)/5-0	0.00	0.20	0.20	0.20	0.20	0.20
C6:PPD333|333-0	0.00	0.00	0.00	0.00	1.00	0.00
C7:PPD333|(333+100)/2-0	0.00	0.00	0.00	0.50	0.50	0.00
C8:PPD333|(333+100+33)/3-0	0.00	0.00	0.33	0.33	0.33	0.00
C9:PPD333|(333+100+33+10)/4-0	0.00	0.25	0.25	0.25	0.25	0.00
C10:PPD100|100-0	0.00	0.00	0.00	1.00	0.00	0.00
C11:PPD100|(100+33)/2-0	0.00	0.00	0.50	0.50	0.00	0.00
C12:PPD100|(100+33+10)/3-0	0.00	0.33	0.33	0.33	0.00	0.00
C13:PPD33|33-0	0.00	0.00	1.00	0.00	0.00	0.00
C14:PPD33|(33+10)/2-0	0.00	0.50	0.50	0.00	0.00	0.00
C15:PPD10|10-0	0.00	1.00	0.00	0.00	0.00	0.00

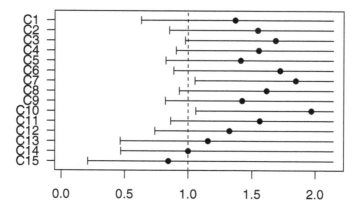

FIGURE 4.2: Ratio-to-control comparisons for downturn protected Williams-type test.

Most contrasts are under H_0 (lower limit smaller than its value of 1). In the alternative is the contrast C10, i.e., assuming a trend up to $100ml/g$ dose as peak point dose (and to a lesser extend contrast C7). But its lower limit 1.06 is rather small; even its point estimator of 1.97 is not above 2-fold rule. A statistically significant partial trend occurs, whereas its biological relevance seems to be questionable. On the other hand, the inappropriate analysis assuming a monotone increasing trend would yield a clear non-significant two-sided p-value of 0.072.

A similar approach denoted as *trimming* was used for BMD estimation for the remaining monotone part of the dose-response relationship [381]. The identification of the NOEAL when downturn effects may occur was recently described [403]. The above downturn-protected Williams test can be extended to a combined test of Dunnett, Williams, and peak-point contrasts (see Section 2.1.2.2). The basic idea is a reasonable compromise between getting information on all interesting inferences and a small multiplicity penalty of simultaneous testing of so many contrasts due to their high correlations. From the perspective of model selection [232] such a complex approach can be recommended for routine use.

4.3 Evaluation of the micronucleus assay as an example for non-parametric tests in small sample size design

Nonparametric tests in toxicology, frequently two-sample Mann–Whitney tests, are the standard approach in toxicology, e.g., for the evaluation of olive tail moments in oocytes [105]. Furthermore, the k-sample Kruskal-Wallis test (sometimes followed by pairwise Wilcoxon-tests) is a common style of evaluation [48, 256]. Already the combination of a global test with pairwise tests may be problematic (see details in Section 2.2.2). Here, the use of nonparametric tests for designs with small sample sizes, such as $n_i = 3$ in the Ames assay or $n_i = 5$ in the *in vivo* micronucleus assay, will be discussed. The n_i are *small* in terms of both power (i.e., power decreases monotonically with smaller n_i), and size (i.e., the concurrent level α is violated). Several tests, such as the Wilcoxon–test, are defined asymptotically and therefore they do not control level α for designs with too small sample sizes. A further complication is the too low power of pre-tests on test condition, such as on a particular distribution, or variance homogeneity; see the discussion on decision tree approaches in Section 1.2.11. Testing for relative effect size represents an interesting alternative (see details in Section 2.1.4) but they control level α only for moderate sample sizes of about $n_i > 10$ [226]. Permutation tests as an alternative can be rather conservative for such designs [192]. The first recommendation is to use designs with not too small sample sizes, e.g., $n_i > 5$ [45]. But this would be a contradiction to some guidelines. The second is to use a t-test (as the best of all bad variants) because it is already defined for a design of $n_1 = 2, n_2 = 1$. The third is the use of permutation tests. As an example, a two-sample design was extracted from the MN data for control and high dose only; see Table 4.2, i.e., small sample sizes with $n_i = 5$ and count data with many ties occur.

Table 4.2: Micronucleus Data as Small Sample Size Two-Sample Example

group	animal	MN
Control	1	4
Control	2	2
Control	3	4
Control	4	2
Control	5	2
D750	16	2
D750	17	4
D750	18	1
D750	19	1
D750	20	0

```
> data("mn", package="SiTuR")
> mn2 <-droplevels(mn[mn$group %in% c("Control","D750"), ])

> tT <-t.test(MN~group, data=mn2, var.equal=TRUE)$p.value
> library("nparcomp")
> relE <-npar.t.test(MN~group, data=mn2, method ="t.app",
+                    info=FALSE)$Analysis$p.Value
```

```
> relP <-npar.t.test(MN~group, data=mn2, method ="permu",
+                      info=FALSE)$Analysis$p.value
> library("coin")
> npA <- pvalue(wilcox_test(MN~group, data=mn2, distribution="asymptotic"))
> npE <- pvalue(wilcox_test(MN~group, data=mn2, distribution="exact"))
```

The large p-value for the two-sided exact (permutation) Wilcoxon–test of 0.206 (in the object **npE**) is not surprising when compared with those of the asymptotic Wilcoxon–test 0.125 (in the object **npA**), the permutation test for relative effects 0.113 (in the object **relP**) and the t-test 0.189 (in the object **tT**). Notice, the use of the t-test for these tied data is problematic, because then five informative different values exist [352]. Already this little example demonstrates how critical two-sample tests for small sample sizes can be. A second problem is the robustness properties of nonparametric tests. Common-used tests, such as the two-sample Wilcoxon or the k-sample Kruskal–Wallis test are problematic for tied data and when variance heterogeneity occurs, particularly for small sample sizes - a not uncommon situation in toxicology (see Section 1.3.3). Statistics for the relative effect size can be used instead [62, 331]. This approach is available in the package **nparcomp** [230] for two-sample comparisons [277], for Dunnett- or Williams-type procedures [228, 229] and as an alternative to the Kruskal–Wallis test as contrast test against the grand mean [227].

The nonparametric proof of hazard approach including a control and several doses is demonstrated in the following by means of the MN data (without positive control).

Table 4.3: Micronucleus Data: Control and Dose Groups

group	animal	MN
Control	1	4
Control	2	2
Control	3	4
Control	4	2
Control	5	2
D188	6	3
D188	7	5
D188	8	7
D188	9	2
D188	10	0
D375	11	5
D375	12	6
D375	13	1
D375	14	4
D375	15	2
D750	16	2
D750	17	4
D750	18	1
D750	19	1
D750	20	0

From Table 4.3 rather small sample sizes and tied values can be seen, and in the boxplots (4.3a) variance heterogeneity is obvious.

The Kruskal–Wallis test is a global test assuming a continuous distributed endpoint with homogeneous variances (see the object KW). As an alternative, a contrast test against the grand mean [227] allows both heterogeneous variances and a discrete distribution for the

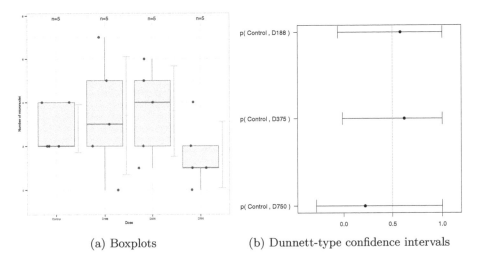

(a) Boxplots   (b) Dunnett-type confidence intervals

FIGURE 4.3: Evaluation of relative effects.

relative effect size (in the object KWp).

```
> library("coin")
> KW <- pvalue(kruskal_test(MN ~ group, data = mnWP,
+        distribution ="asymptotic"), method = "single-step" )
> library("nparcomp")
> aveRE <-nparcomp(MN~group, data=mnWP, type="AVE", asy.method = "mult.t",
+                info = FALSE, correlation=TRUE)$Analysis$p.Value
> KWp <-min(aveRE)
```

The p-values of both approaches differ slightly: $p_{KW} = 0.333$ vs. $p_{contrastGM} = 0.249$. While the Kruskal–Wallis test assumes continuous data and homogeneity of variances and provides only a single p-value on global heterogeneity, the multiple contrast test allows discrete data, heterogeneous variances, and provides individual inferences (where the global p-value is the minimum of all elementary p-values). Moreover, it allows one-sided tests. However, it is an asymptotic approach and therefore requires not too small sample sizes, such as $n_i > 10$.

Instead of a global test, the use of Dunnett-type approaches can be recommended (see details in Section 2.1.1). Either a permutation version of the Steel test (object SteelA) can be used (using the package coin) or an asymptotic procedure for relative effect sizes (object SteelRE) (using the package nparcomp) can be used.

```
> library("coin")
> SteelA <- oneway_test(MN ~ group, data = mnWP,
+ ytrafo = function(data) trafo(data, numeric_trafo = rank),
+ xtrafo = function(data) trafo(data, factor_trafo = function(x)
+ model.matrix(~x - 1) %*% t(contrMat(table(x), "Dunnett"))),
+ teststat = "maximum", distribution ="asymptotic", alternative="greater")
> SteelAp <-pvalue(SteelA, method = "single-step")
> library("nparcomp")
> SteelRE <-nparcomp(MN~group, data=mnWP, type="Dunnett",
+          asy.method = "mult.t",alternative = "greater",
+     plot.simci =FALSE, info = FALSE, correlation=TRUE)$Analysis$p.Value
```

The *p*-values differ not substantial, e.g., for the comparison of the low dose against control for the permutative Steel test with 0.333 and for relative effects with 0.712.

The better way of presentation is the use of simultaneous confidence limits for relative effect size in Figure 4.3b. All confidence intervals contain the value of the null-hypothesis of 0.5, i.e., no changes in the number of micronuclei occur in this bioassay.

4.4   Evaluation of the SHE assay using trend tests on proportions

Syrian hamster embryo (SHE) cells have been used in a clonal cell transformation assay to assess the carcinogenic potential of chemicals [383]. The primary endpoint is the number of morphologically transformed (MT) colonies per total number of colonies scored for each treatment group. Commonly pooled data from multiple trials were used. By means of a goodness-of-fit test on control data it was previously confirmed that the data across independent trials are consistent with the binomial distribution and hence pooling is valid [235]. These proportions are evaluated by both pairwise comparisons between the dose groups and the negative control using one-sided Fisher's exact tests (each at level α) and the Cochran–Armitage trend test in the original publication [211]. Scoring 1000 colonies per treatment group with an average control transformation frequency of 0.4% allows for a 4- to 5-fold increase in transformation to be detected as significant at the 0.05 level with a power of 80% [202]. The compound is considered positive if it causes a statistically significant increase in at least two dose levels by Fisher's exact test or a significant increase in one dose with a statistically significant Cochran–Armitage trend test at level $\alpha = 0.05$ with either a 24-h or a 7-day exposure to the test chemical [202]. The data can be summarized in a 2-by-k contingency table. As an example the table data for an SHE-assay on anilazine from Table 2 [211] are presented in Table 4.4.

Table 4.4: Raw Data of the Anilazine SHE Bioassay

	control	D10	D20	D35	D50
MT	5	0	3	2	20
noMT	2727	1555	1478	1344	1409

From a statistical perspective, the proportions in this contingency table are small: from 0.0018 in the control up to 0.0140 in the high dose and the number of scored colonies is large from 1344 to 2727. For these data the following questions arise when using pairwise Fisher's exact tests and Cochran–Armitage trend test [202]: i) are inconsistent results possible when using pairwise tests after a significant trend test?, ii) is Fisher exact test appropriate although known to be conservative?, iii) are tests for the difference to control appropriate or should ratio-to-control tests (namely for relative risk (RR) or for odds ratio (RR)) used instead, because as relevance criterion a k-fold increase is used? iv) are one-sided tests for an increase appropriate? v) are confidence limits for RR or OR appropriate?, and vi) should the overdispersion between replicated trials be taken into account?

4.4.1 The Cochran–Armitage trend test for proportions

Commonly, as trend test for proportions the Cochran–Armitage test [31] is used. This test is a Wald test for a linear logistic regression model and therefore sensitive for near-to-linear shapes of the dose-response relationship. Its data model is a 2-by-k table, i.e., overdispersion for replicated proportion (e.g., between animals) is ignored. An asymptotic, an approximate, and an exact version exist [192] as well as a one-sided and a two-sided version (although a restriction to an ordered alternative without a directional restriction is hard to imagine). No confidence intervals are available and the effect size is a hard-to-interpret slope. Challenging problems are the optimal choice of scores [130] and the adjustment against covariates. It is a quadratic form of a linear by linear association test [309], a permutation test on the correlation between a binary endpoint and a covariate [192, 194].

The standard CA-trend test is defined for the concurrent dose scores. An alternative is the use of equidistant scores, denoted linear-by-linear-association test. In these data a specific trend exists where only an increase in the high dose (D50) exists (in the object CA) and therefore a maximum-type contrast test with the dose scores $0, 0, 0, 0, 1$ reveals the smallest p-value (in the object lin0. Not surprisingly, a simple heterogeneity test (without assuming any trend in the object Hetero) reveals even a smaller p-value than the standard CA-trend test because the latter is defined for a linear shape; see Table 4.5.

```
> library("coin")
> library("xtable")
> Hetero <-independence_test(an ~ group, data =ana, teststat = "quad")
> HeterogeneityTest <-pvalue(Hetero, method = "single-step")
> CA <-independence_test(an ~ Group, data = ana, teststat = "quad")
> LinearLinearAssociationTest <-pvalue(CA, method = "single-step")
> CAdose <-independence_test(an ~ Group, data = ana, teststat = "quad",
+               scores = list(Group = c(0, 10, 20, 35, 50)))
> CochranArmitageTest <-pvalue(CAdose, method = "single-step")
> lin0 <-independence_test(an ~ Group, data = ana, teststat = "maximum",
+               distribution = "asymptotic",
+               scores = list(Group = c(0, 0, 0, 0, 1)))
> ContrastTest <-pvalue(lin0, method = "single-step")
> pvalsCA <-as.data.frame(rbind(HeterogeneityTest,
+       LinearLinearAssociationTest, CochranArmitageTest, ContrastTest))
```

Table 4.5: p-Values for Different Tests

	p-value
HeterogeneityTest	0.00000000003
LinearLinearAssociationTest	0.00000021141
CochranArmitageTest	0.00000002463
ContrastTest	0.00000000000

A further modification is a step-down closure principle procedure. Using an *a priori* importance by means of a monotone alternative, a simple step-down procedure can be performed: if $test^{CA}_{C,D_1,...D_k}$ significant at level α test $test^{CA}_{C,D_1,...D_{k-1}}$ (and conditional downwards up to $test^{CA}_{C,D_1}$, otherwise stop [171, 258, 178]. This allows the identification of the lowest significant dose level as long as the monotonicity assumption is fulfilled. For the above example the code is simple.

```
> library("coin")
> CAdose <-independence_test(an ~ Group, data = ana, teststat = "quad",
+                       scores = list(Group = c(0, 10, 20, 35, 50)))
> pCAD <-pvalue(CAdose, method = "single-step")
> ana4 <-droplevels(ana[ana$Group!="D50", ])
> CAdose4 <-independence_test(an ~ Group, data = ana4, teststat = "quad",
+                       scores = list(Group = c(0, 10, 20, 35)))
> pCAD4 <-pvalue(CAdose4, method = "single-step")
```

Whereas the global CA-trend test is significant (p-value of 2.46×10^{-8}), already the trend test up to dose D35 is no more significant (p-value of 0.994). i.e., the trend is supported by the highest dose only.

4.4.2   Trend tests followed by pairwise tests

The problems arising with pairwise tests (each at level α) conditional or unconditional after a global test (such as ANOVA) are discussed in Section 1.2.11 in detail. A special case is one-sided pairwise tests following a significant trend test. Three claims may be intended: i) to detect a downturn effect at high doses even when the trend test is not significant, ii) to identify the minimum significant dose, and iii) to characterize the specific pattern of the dose-response relationship. This first case is discussed in Section 2.1.2.2, the second in 7.3, the third in 7.1. The question arises which two-sample tests for proportions should be used (see also Section 1.3.4). The common Fisher's exact test can be rather conservative for small sample sizes [83] and should be avoided particularly in toxicology (causing too high false negative errors). A χ^2 test can be used when the smallest expected cell count is $np > 1$ [68], i.e., already for spontaneous rates of 10% and sample size of 10. One-sided confidence limits represent a specific problem, particularly for the three effect sizes (risk difference RD, risk ratio RR, and odds ratio OR), specifically whether to account for extra-binomial variability or not [187]. From the above example data a 2-by-2 table data containing control and the high dose was selected. Three types of small-sample size lower confidence limits were estimated for using the package `pairwiseCI` for RD, RR and OR:

```
> library("pairwiseCI")
> Difference <-Prop.diff(x=cont, y=D50, CImethod="AC",
+                    alternative="less")$conf.int[2]
> RR <-          Prop.ratio(x=cont, y=D50,  CImethod="MOVER",
+                    alternative="less")$conf.int[2]
> OR <-          Prop.or(x=cont, y=D50, CImethod="Woolf",
+                    alternative="less")$conf.int[2]
```

Table 4.6: Lower Limits for Small-Sample Size Pairwise Comparison of Proportions

	Lower confidence limit
Difference	-0.007
RR	0.295
OR	0.306

After the significant trend test, all pairwise tests vs. control are performed in the above example (4.4.1]). Only the highest dose is significantly increased with respect to control. The upper confidence limits for the effect size risk difference (RD) using the asymptotic Wald-type interval after adding one pseudo-observation to each cell [22] can be seen in Table 4.6 (notice the value of H_0 is 0). Furthermore, both for the relative risk (RR) using the asymptotic variance estimate recovery for ratios [18] and the odds ratio (OR) using the asymptotic adjusted Woolf-type confidence interval after adding 0.5 to each cell count [234] are reported in Table 4.6 (notice the value of H_0 is 1). Notice, the related test decisions are not necessarily compatible, summarizing, a somewhat specific shape of a trend in toxicological risk assessment.

4.4.3 Evaluation using Dunnett-type procedure for proportions

The common-used approach in toxicology for comparisons of several treatment or dose groups versus control is the Dunnett [102] procedure. Notice, Dunnett's procedure controls the familywise error rate (FWER) which causes an increase of the false negative decision rate compared with two-sample tests each at level α. Here, we use a Dunnett-type procedure for proportions [347] namely: i) for the risk difference (RD), ii) the risk ratio (RR), or iii) the odds ratio (OR) (see for details Section 2.1.5). For the above anilazine SHE bioassay example let us focus here on odds ratios and their simultaneous confidence intervals, or more appropriate the one-sided lower limits. This can be performed by means of the generalized linear model (GLM) (and the logit link function `family= binomial(link="logit")`) (see Section 2.1.5.1 for details) or taking the small sample behavior into account by the Woolf adjustment (see Section 2.1.5.3 for details). Notice, the functions glm and binomORci use differently defined responder-to-nonresponder data, therefore in the first codeline the reversed variable (**ana$anrev**) is calculated and used in **glm()**.

```
> library("multcomp")
> ana$anrev <- factor(ana$an, levels=rev(levels(ana$an)))
> fitORrev <- glm(anrev ~ group, data=ana, family= binomial(link="logit"))
> ciORrev <- glht(fitORrev, linfct = mcp(group = "Dunnett"),
+                 alternative="greater")
> ciorrev <- exp(confint(ciORrev)$confint)
> library("MCPAN")
> withA<-anaTab[1,1:5]
> totalA <-anaTab[2,1:5]+anaTab[1,1:5]
> ciorA1 <-binomORci(n=totalA, x=withA, alternative="greater",
+                 method="Woolf", type="Dunnett")
> ciorA0 <-binomORci(n=totalA, x=withA, alternative="greater",
+                 method="GLM", type="Dunnett")
> ORs <-round(ciorA1$estimate,2)
> lORglm <-signif(ciorrev[,"lwr"],2)
> lORwoolf <-signif(ciorA1$conf.int[,"lower"],2)
```

Both approaches are compared for the anilazine SHE data example, whereas in Table 4.7 the lower limits do not differ too much. Again, only a significant increase of the micronuclei proportion in the highest dose can be stated because the lower confidence limits are > 1 (the value of H_0 for OR's). These results can be quite different when using small sample sizes data and near-to-zero proportions occur in the control. Similarly, Williams-type tests can be performed; see Section 2.1.6.3 for details.

Table 4.7: Odds Ratio with GLM-Style and Woolf-Adjusted Lower Limits

	OR	lowerCI-GLM	lowerCI-Woolf
D10 / control	0.16	0.00	0.00
D20 / control	1.17	0.22	0.26
D35 / control	0.92	0.13	0.17
D50 / control	7.21	2.60	2.50

4.5   Evaluation of the *in vivo* micronucleus assay as an example of the analysis of proportions taking overdispersion into account

The primary endpoint in the *in vivo* micronucleus assay according to the OECD guideline No. 474 [288] is the number of micronucleated erythocytes (MN) per a certain number of scored polychromatic erythrocytes (PCE), per animal. Therefore, binomial proportions MN/PCE can be used as endpoint. Two designs can be distinguished: i) one with almost constant number of commonly 2000 scored cells (see the 1-phenylethanol bioassay example [110]) and their analysis with counts (see details in Section 4.6), or ii) data with a rather different number of scored cells; see the micronucleus assay with 5-(4-Nitroglycerin)-2,4-pentadien-1-al (NPPD) on the peripheral blood of B6C3F1 mice using the standard NTP protocol [7], where the NPPD data set can be found in Table 4.8.

```
> data("np", package="SiTuR")
> np$Risk <-np$PCE-np$MN
```

Table 4.8: NPPD Dataset

Dose	Animal	PCE	MN	Risk
Control	1	15154	22	15132
Control	10	11063	14	11049
Control	2	10384	19	10365
Control	3	12094	9	12085
Control	4	11577	16	11561
...	...	...	...	...
D3	56	9760	46	9714
D3	57	9970	53	9917
D3	58	9766	63	9703
D3	59	12340	63	12277
D3	60	9970	32	9938

The individual animal is the experimental unit; it is randomized, it is treated in this micronucleus assay. Therefore, the variability between the animals should be taken into account in principle. Pooling the number of MN over the animals of a group, as proposed by [213], results in too liberal decisions and cannot be recommended. This between-animal variability can be considered for counts by means of a quasi-Poisson model, where a dispersion parameter is estimated from the data, characterizing this between animals variability [297]; see details in Section 4.6. For binomial proportions with overdispersion a mixed model (see Section 2.1.5.4.1) or the quasi-binomial or negative binomial model in the GLM can be used;

see below. A second statistical aspect is the use of confidence intervals for an appropriate effects size, such as the relative risk (RR) or the odds ratio (OR).

Using the link-function `logit`, the effect size odds ratio (OR) is used and additionally by means of the argument `family=quasibinomial(link="logit")` the overdispersion between the proportions is taken into account.

```
> fitqbPair <-glm(cbind(MN, Risk) ~ Dose, data=np,
+                 family=quasibinomial(link="logit"))
> DispP <-round(summary(fitqbPair)$dispersion, 2)
> library("multcomp")
> MCPPair <- glht(fitqbPair, linfct = mcp(Dose = "Dunnett"),
+                 alternative="greater")
> fitbPair <-glm(cbind(MN, Risk) ~ Dose, data=np,
+                 family=binomial(link="logit"))
> MCPPb <- glht(fitbPair, linfct = mcp(Dose = "Dunnett"),
+               alternative="greater")
```

The estimated dispersion parameter of 2.67 indicates a substantial between-animal variability. On the other hand, when using the family `binomial` the number of MN and PCE are pooled for each animal and just a single proportion per treatment group is used.

Table 4.9: Lower Confidence Limits for the Odds Ratios against Control in the NPPD Example

	OR	lower_quasiBin	lower_Bin
D0.03 - Control	1.38	1.04	1.16
D0.1 - Control	1.01	0.74	0.83
D0.3 - Control	1.28	0.96	1.07
D1 - Control	1.68	1.28	1.43
D3 - Control	3.65	2.85	3.14

Not surprisingly those confidence limits in Table 4.9 ignoring the overdispersion (`lower_Bin`) are falsely more in the alternative than those taking the overdispersion into account (`lowerquasi_Bin`) ; even with a qualitatively different conclusion for the dose D0.3 (non-significant vs. significant).

4.6 Evaluation of the *in vivo* micronucleus assay as an example of the analysis of counts taking overdispersion into account

Overdispersed proportions are used when the numbers of scored cells are different per animal (see Section 4.5) whereas overdispersed counts when they are almost constant. As an example a micronucleus assay on three doses of phenylethanol, together with a negative control and a positive control [110] was selected; see the raw data in Table 4.10 and in the boxplots in Figure 4.4.

```
> data("mn", package="SiTuR")
```

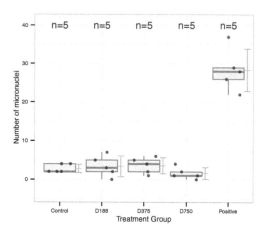

FIGURE 4.4: Boxplots micronucleus assay on phenylethanol.

Again, the between-animal variability should be considered. Generalized Poisson distributions can be used, where the negative binomial model was recommended for count data [395]. Several algorithms for fitting count data are available [416]. Simple is the function `glm.nb` in the package `MASS` [384]. In the framework of a generalized linear model, counts can be modeled on the log scale, assuming a Poisson distribution, where the variance is constrained to be completely determined by the mean $V(\mu) = \mu$. Because the assumption of a variance determined completely by the mean may be not reliable, one can fit a negative binomial model with variance function $V(\mu) = \mu + \phi\mu^2$. The estimated dispersion parameter $\hat{\phi}$ will be small, if the data are near to Poisson distributed, and accounts for overdispersion if it is increasing.

```
> library("multcomp")
> library("MASS")
> mna <-droplevels(mn[mn$group!="Positive",])
> fitnbN <- glm.nb(MN ~ group, data=mna)
> fitqpN <- glm(MN ~ group, data=mna, family=quasipoisson(link="log"))
> dispDu <-summary(fitqpN)$dispersion
> DuMNH  <- glht(fitnbN, linfct = mcp(group ="Dunnett"),
+          alternative = "greater")
> DuMNqH <- glht(fitqpN, linfct = mcp(group ="Dunnett"),
+          alternative="greater")
> fitp <- glm(MN ~ group, data=mna, family=poisson(link="log"))
> DuMp <- glht(fitp, linfct = mcp(group ="Dunnett"), alternative="greater")
```

In the example the dispersion was estimated to 1.3, i.e., the MN counts are near to Poisson distributed.

Alternatives to account for extra variation are quasi-likelihood methods where the model can be fitted under the assumption $V(\mu) = \rho\mu$. A value of ρ larger than 1 indicates overdispersion. The estimated dispersion parameter in the example has a value of 1.3, i.e., the variance of the estimated parameters in the quasi-Poisson model is only a little larger

Table 4.10: Raw Data of the Micronucleus Assay on Phenylethanol.

group	animal	MN
Control	1	4
Control	2	2
Control	3	4
Control	4	2
Control	5	2
D188	6	3
D188	7	5
D188	8	7
D188	9	2
D188	10	0
D375	11	5
D375	12	6
D375	13	1
D375	14	4
D375	15	2
D750	16	2
D750	17	4
D750	18	1
D750	19	1
D750	20	0
Positive	21	26
Positive	22	28
Positive	22	22
Positive	23	37
Positive	24	29

Table 4.11: Point Estimate and Three Types of Lower Confidence Limits

	OR	LowerLimit_negbin	LowerLimit_quasiPoisson	LowerLimit_Poisson
D188 - Control	1.21	0.56	0.52	0.58
D375 - Control	1.29	0.60	0.56	0.62
D750 - Control	0.57	0.22	0.20	0.23

than in the Poisson model. It is the same Poisson model but with the dispersion parameter being estimated *posthoc*, after fitting the model. These small differences can also be seen for the estimated Dunnett-type lower limits for the three models: negative binomial, quasi-Poisson and Poisson in Table 4.11. Notice, these estimated confidence limits are asymptotic only [189]. An alternative is to use the generalized mixed model with Poisson link function. Similar confidence limits for the OR are given in Table 4.12.

```
> library("multcomp")
> library("lme4")
> fitmM <- glmer(MN ~ group + (1|animal), data=mna,
+         family=poisson(link="log"))
> mMP <-glht(fitmM, linfct = mcp(group = "Dunnett"), alternative="greater")
```

In this particular example all four approaches (negative binomial, quasi-Poisson, Poisson distribution, and mixed model for Poisson-distributed endpoints) reveal similar lower confidence limits with the general conclusion: no increase in either dose with respect to control. However, in this example the between-animal variability was small. For general recommendation further work is needed, particularly for designs with small sample sizes and dose-dependent overdispersion.

Table 4.12: Lower Confidence Limits for Generalized Linear Mixed Model

	LowerLimit_mixedPoisson
D188 - Control	0.56
D375 - Control	0.60
D750 - Control	0.22

4.7 Evaluation of HET-MN assay for an example of transformed count data

Although count data are common in mutagenicity assays, a specific problem occurs when zero or near-to-zero counts in the control are observed, particularly when small sample sizes are used. As an alternative to modeling overdispersed counts in the generalized linear (mixed) model (GLMM; see Section 4.6), data transformation can be used. Transforming count data into pseudo-normally distributed endpoints with homogeneous variances was used for cell transformation assays [280, 166], the Ames fluctuation assay [318] and Hen's egg micronucleus assay [179]. Different transformations are available, whereas for overdispersed near-to-zero counts x_{ij} the simple Freeman–Tukey (FT) root transformation [118] can be recommended: $X_{ij}^{\text{FT}} = \sqrt{X_{ij}} + \sqrt{X_{ij} + 1}$, where i represents the group index and j the subject index [135]. As example a Hen's egg micronucleus assay [179] (1st dataset) was used; see the raw with the FT-transformed data (ft) in Table 4.13. The transformed data are simply analyzed by the standard Dunnett test.

```
> library("multcomp")
> d1$ft   <- sqrt(d1$MN)+ sqrt(d1$MN+1)       # FT transformation
> f1      <- lm(ft ~ Dose, data=d1)          # fit linear model
> g1D     <- glht(f1, linfct=mcp(Dose="Dunnett" ), alternative="greater")
> Dun     <- summary(g1D)$test$pvalues       # FT-Dunnett  p-values
```

The disadvantage of a hard-to-interpret effect size of the difference of transformed values can be circumvented by reporting just the p-values of a test on transformed data. Raw means should be reported and stated that the p-values are based on transformed data. For the simple example the related Dunnett-type p-values are 0.934, 0.773, 0.009 for comparisons of the negative control against low, medium, and high dose, i.e., a significant increase of the MN with respect to control occurs in the high dose group only.

4.8 Evaluation of cell transformation assay for an example of near-to-zero counts in the control

In several toxicological assays endpoints of pathological response are used, such as number of tumors or number of micronuclei (see the endpoint classification in Section 1.2.6). For theses endpoints a specific problem may arise, namely zero or near-to-zero counts or proportions in the control, particularly when small sample sizes are used. Several statistical approaches

Table 4.13: Hen's Egg Micronucleus Assay Data

Dose	MN	ft
NC	2	3.15
NC	2	3.15
NC	4	4.24
NC	0	1.00
NC	3	3.73
NC	2	3.15
D1	0	1.00
D1	1	2.41
D1	7	5.47
D1	0	1.00
D1	0	1.00
D1	1	2.41
D2	1	2.41
D2	8	5.83
D2	2	3.15
D2	2	3.15
D2	0	1.00
D2	1	2.41
D3	3	3.73
D3	14	7.61
D3	28	10.68
D3	19	8.83
D3	2	3.15
D3	6	5.10

can be used, here we demonstrate a profile likelihood approach and the FT-transformation, already discussed in the previous Section 4.7.

4.8.1 Profile likelihood

As example using count data, the cell transformation assay [166] was used (see the boxplots in Figure 4.5). The number of transformed foci is used as a single primary endpoints and a one-way layout with a control and several concentrations is used. From the boxplots in Figure 4.5 the specific problem becomes clear: near-to-zero counts in the control. When designs with small sample sizes are used and the estimates approach the border of the parameter space, likelihood profiles based signed likelihood root statistics can improve the properties of simultaneous confidence intervals [124] - even in situations when Wald-type intervals are uninformative. Specific applications are small sample size bioassays with near-to-zero count data in the control.

```
> data("cta", package="mcprofile")
> cta$Dose <- factor(cta$conc, levels=unique(cta$conc))
```

The related package mcprofile allows a rather simple use of this new approach; see the related confidence interval in Figure 4.6.

```
> library("mcprofile")
> ctaGLM <- glm(foci ~ Dose, data=cta, family=poisson(link="log"))
> library("multcomp")
> CM <- contrMat(table(cta$Dose), type="Dunnett")
> mpCI <- mcprofile(ctaGLM, CM)
```

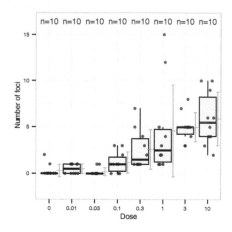

FIGURE 4.5: Boxplots for cell transformation assay.

> *plot(confint(mpCI), hlines=1)*

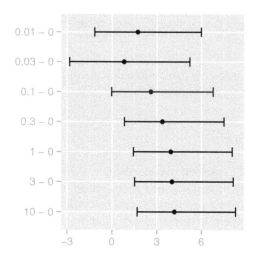

FIGURE 4.6: Dunnett-type profile likelihood intervals for cell transformation assay.

For all doses above 0.3 the lower confidence limits are larger than 1.0 and hence a significant increase can be concluded.

4.8.2   FT-transformation

As described in the previous Section 4.7 a Dunnett-type test on FT-transformed endpoint is simple:

```
> library("multcomp")
> cta$FT <- sqrt(cta$foci)+ sqrt(cta$foci+1)
> FT1     <- lm(FT ~ Dose, data=cta)
> FTD    <- glht(FT1, linfct=mcp(Dose="Dunnett"), alternative="greater")
> FTDun    <- summary(FTD)$test$pvalues
```

The multiplicity-adjusted p-values in the object `FTDun` reveal a similar decision as the Dunnett-type profile likelihood intervals in Figure 4.6: all doses greater than 0.1 reveal a significant increase in number of foci.

4.8.3 Zero-inflated Poisson model

Near-to-zero counts can also be modeled as zero-inflated Poisson variables ([416]). In the framework of generalized additive models, the package `gamlss` is available [361] where a family argument `ZIP` (stands for zero-inflated Poisson by an extra parameter for describing the excess zeros) can be used:

```
> library("multcomp")
> library("gamlss")
> library("BSagri")
> ctaZIP  <- gamlss(foci ~ Dose, data=cta, family=ZIP)
```

GAMLSS-RS iteration 1: Global Deviance = 267.1467 GAMLSS-RS iteration 2: Global Deviance = 266.9497 GAMLSS-RS iteration 3: Global Deviance = 266.9496

```
> ctaP <-glht(ctaZIP, linfct=mcp(Dose="Dunnett"), alternative="greater")
> ctaS <-summary(ctaP)
```

The related multiplicity-adjusted p-values are in Table 4.14.

Table 4.14: Adjusted p-Values for Zero-Inflated Poisson Model

	Comparison vs. control	p-value
1	0.01 - 0	0.55223
2	0.03 - 0	0.91473
3	0.1 - 0	0.03423
4	0.3 - 0	0.00016
5	1 - 0	0.00000
6	3 - 0	0.00002
7	10 - 0	0.00000

Again, all doses above 0.1 reveal a significant increase in number of foci. Although for a pathological endpoint zeros are common especially for the control group, no recommendation for a particular method (of the above three or even alternatives) can be given because too little is known up to now of their behavior (size, power) particularly in small sample sizes and only zeros in the control. More research on this topic is needed.

4.9   Evaluation of the LLNA as an example for k-fold rule

Standardized by the OECD guideline no. 429 [286], the local lymph node assay (LLNA) provides an alternative method for identifying skin sensitizing compounds. At least three doses of the test substance D_i and a negative control C are used in a randomized one-way with at least five animals per treatment group as randomized unit. Several endpoints are used, such as cellularity or lymph node weight. From a statistical perspective, we assume any continuous endpoint, measured on each animal j as a univariate endpoint y_{ij} in a design including a negative control and some treatment groups D_i. Based on the relative k-fold relevance criteria, we propose a statistical approach using confidence limits for ratio-to-control comparisons without a monotonic dose-response assumption. For two mice strains (NMRI and BALB/c) the two endpoints cellularity (cell) and lymph node weight (lnw) were measured in a control and three doses ($D_{low}, D_{med}, D_{xtr}$) for six animals each [180].

```
> data("vor", package="SiTuR")
```

The boxplots in Figure 4.7 indicate some increasing effect, approximate symmetric distributions, mild variance heterogeneity (notice $n_i = 6$!), and some extreme values.

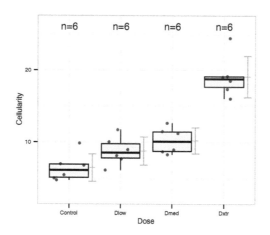

FIGURE 4.7: Boxplots BALB/c cellularity.

A positive response is defined as k-fold increase of $k = 1.55$ for cellularity in BALB/c mice based on an interlaboratory study [104]. A relative change threshold is used as relevance criterion, analogously to the k-fold rule in the Ames assays [70]. Therefore, the ratio-to-control version of the Dunnett procedure is used assuming that cellularity is normally distributed with homogeneous variances [95, 97]. Alternatively, confidence limits for ratio-to-control using the naive log-transformation are estimated to compare both approaches (see Section 2.1.3).

Table 4.15 shows no significant increase for the low dose, statistically significant but biologically non-relevant increase in the medium dose (because the lower limit is < 1.55), and both significant and relevant increase in the high dose for the primary endpoint cellularity (and slightly different results for the log-transformation approach).

```
> library("mratios")
> normratio <-sci.ratio(cell_BALB~group, data=vor, method="Plug",
+                       type="Dunnett", alternative="greater")
> library("multcomp")
> lcell <-log(vor$cell_BALB)
> mylmod <-lm(lcell~group, data=vor)
> myci <-confint(glht(mylmod, linfct=mcp(group="Dunnett"),
+        alternative="greater"))
> myconf <-exp(myci$confint) # naive log normal
```

Table 4.15: Lower Confidence Limits for Ratio-to-Control Comparisons either Using Estimated Ratios Directly and via a Naive Log Transformation

	normal	log-normal
Dlow/Control	0.96	1.05
Dmed/Control	1.14	1.24
Dxtr/Control	2.25	2.33

4.10 Evaluation of the HET-MN assay using historical control data

Historical controls can be used directly for a test decision or the estimation of reference values, particularly available for proportions, such as tumor rates [215] (see Section 3.3.2 for details). For continuous data such an approach is even more complicated. We use as historical controls the example data of the 24 runs in lab B [179]; see Figure 4.8.

```
> data("dH", package="SiTuR")
```

Following the US FDA recommendation [14]: *"...the concurrent control group is always the most appropriate and important in testing drug related increases in tumor rates ... as long as the concurrent control data are within the range of historical control data"* a two-step approach was proposed [179]. First we check whether the concurrent control is within a normal range of the historical controls. For FT-transformed historical data (see Section 4.7) a simple 2σ interval can be recommended [21], which does not depend on the number of historical NCs (n_{histNC}).

In our example (see Section 4.7) the mean of the concurrent control of 3.07 is outside the normal range of $[1.23, 2.35]$. Therefore in a second step the mean of the concurrent control is replaced by the mean of the historical control (MwHist) as a known constant. The motivation for the simplified approach is the independence of the number of historical runs (this should not influence a decision). Its disadvantage is ignoring the variation between and within the runs [204].

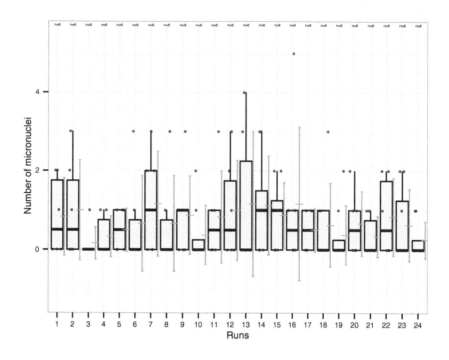

FIGURE 4.8: Historical MN data.

```
> # Williams-type procedure against historical control mean
> library("multcomp")
> n        <- table(d1$Dose)              # Sample sizes for each group
> cmatrix <- contrMat(n, type="Williams")[,-1] # contrast mat w/o NC
> da       <- droplevels(subset(d1, Dose != "NC")) # omit conc NC
> fa       <- lm(ft ~ Dose - 1, data=da)   # fit reduced linear model
> gaW      <- glht(fa, linfct=cmatrix, rhs=MwHist, alternative="greater")
> histWil <- summary(gaW)$test$pvalues
>
> # Williams-type procedure against concurrent control
> fb       <- lm(ft ~ Dose, data=d1)       # fit complete linear model
> gbW      <- glht(fb, linfct=mcp(Dose="Williams"), alternative="greater")
> Wil      <- summary(gbW)$test$pvalues
> hw <-cbind(Wil, histWil)
```

Table 4.16: Williams Test Using Concurrent or Historical Control Means

	Concurrent control	Historical control
1	0.007	0.000
2	0.085	0.000
3	0.272	0.001

Because in the example the concurrent control is much larger than the historical control, the *p*-values for the Williams test using the historical mean are considerably smaller; see Table 4.16.

4.11 Evaluation of a micronucleus assay taking the positive control into account

The use of positive controls in toxicology is quite common (almost 1388 citations in WebSci October 1, 2014), particularly in mutagenicity assays [153]. However, their use in statistical evaluation is rare. First, different positive control values are used to estimate the positive predictive value (respective sensitivity) of new assays [112]. Second, the sensitivity of a single assay can be claimed by a significant pre-test between positive and negative control $\mu_{C+} - \mu_{C-}$ [150]. Third, the positive control can be used to determine the biological relevance of a statistically significant effect (previously tested against negative control). Relevance can be concluded when the sample distribution of a dose group falls within the region of positive control response [207], whereas no statistical test was proposed. Fourth, a non-inferiority test can be used or more rigorously the adjusted effect size $\frac{\mu_{D_i} - \mu_{C-}}{\mu_{C+} - \mu_{C-}}$ [143] in the proof of safety. For the micronucleus data of [20] (see Figure 4.9) these approaches are demonstrated in the following.

```
> data("Mutagenicity", package="mratios")
> Muta <- Mutagenicity
> Muta$Treatment <- factor(Muta$Treatment, levels=c("Vehicle","Hydro30",
+                  "Hydro50","Hydro75","Hydro100","Cyclo25"))
```

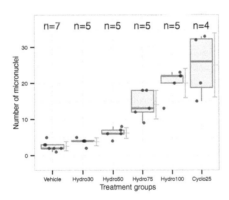

FIGURE 4.9: Micronucleus data including a positive control.

To keep the analysis simple, we assume approximate normal distributed errors for this endpoint (no zeros, values between 1 and 33) and focusing on Dunnett-type ratio-to-control inference:

```
> library("mratios")
> MutaPM <-droplevels(Mutagenicity[Mutagenicity$Treatment
+                          %in% c("Cyclo25", "Vehicle"), ])
> sens <-t.test.ratio(MN~Treatment, data=MutaPM, alternative="greater",
+                  var.equal=FALSE)
```

First, the proof of sensitivity is performed by a two-sample test positive against negative control (allowing heterogeneous variances) in the object **sens**. The *p*-value of 0.007 reveals a clear assay sensitivity.

```
> library("mratios")
> MutaN <-droplevels(Mutagenicity[Mutagenicity$Treatment !="Cyclo25", ])
> du2C <-simtest.ratioVH(MN~Treatment, data=MutaN,
+       alternative="greater",  type = "Dunnett", base = 5)$p.value.adj
```

Second, the Dunnett-type *p*-values for the k-fold increases of the dose groups vs. negative control in the object du2C are 0.0054555, 0.1730208, 0.0054601, 0.0012971 for k-fold increase versus control for 30, 50, 75 and 100 mg/kg, i.e., all doses $> 30mg$ are significantly increased.

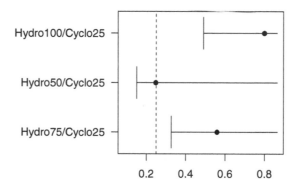

FIGURE 4.10: One-sided lower confidence limits for ratio-to-positive control.

In a third step for these significant doses the question will be answered which of these doses is to some extent non-inferior with respect to the positive control. In Figure 4.10 an arbitrary threshold of 25% is used. Hence, 100 and 75 mg/kg reveal a significant increase with respect to negative control AND a relevant effect, i.e., at least 25% of the positive control.

The adjusted effect size $\frac{\mu_{D_i} - \mu_{C-}}{\mu_{C+} - \mu_{C-}}$ represents the ratio between the concurrent mutagenic effect to the maximum possible effect (given an appropriate compound as positive control in an appropriate dose).

A proof of safety approach is shown in Figure 4.11 where the upper confidence limits for these ratios are compared with an arbitrarily chosen tolerable threshold of 25%, i.e., the 30 mg/kg dose can be assumed as safe, all higher doses cannot.

4.12   Evaluation of the Comet assay as an example for mixing distribution

The Comet assay is a short-term genotoxicity test to detect DNA, damaging compounds where free loops of DNA form comet-shaped structures in gel electrophoresis. Several parameters are derived, such as tail length, moment or intensity [399]. Two specific problems occur from a statistical perspective: i) For *in vivo* studies a hierarchical design

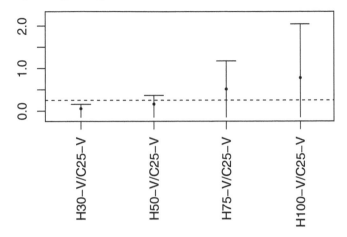

FIGURE 4.11: One-sided upper confidence limits for ratio-to-positive control.

treatment ⊃ *animal* ⊃ *organ* ⊃ *sample* ⊃ *slide* ⊃ *cell* exists and the variability between these items should be modeled using a related mixed model (see also Section 5), ii) the distribution of the endpoints is neither symmetric nor uni-modal, e.g., the % tail DNA in liver is extreme skewed [247]. Therefore, [399] found that the use of log-transformed data is appropriate for the tail moment and the 90th percentile, capturing the upper tail of the distribution, performs well for the tail length [106]. Furthermore, [385] used a mixed model for log-transformed data. As a data example the tail intensities for liver in each 5 animals, 2 samples and each 50 cells is used here [276].

```
> data("TIComet", package="SiTuR")
```

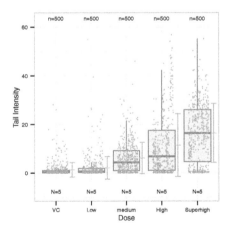

FIGURE 4.12: Boxplots for tail intensities in Comet assay.

The boxplots in Figure 4.12 show dose-dependent skewness and bimodality and the between-animal variability. Four methods are used here [125]: i) responder analysis using a 90th percentile cutpoint estimated from the control group, ii) log-transformation of the tail intensities, iii) responder analysis estimated from a bimodal normal mixing distribution, and

iv) inference on responding animals only. The between-animals and between-samples variability is modeled by means of a mixed model or a generalized linear model assuming
overdispersion.

First, the tail intensities are dichotomized by the 90th percentile cutpoint from the control (object `cutpoint`). Per animal a proportion exists and therefore a between-animals
variability exists, see Table 4.17

```
> subTI <- subset(TIComet, Treatment == "VC")
> cutpoint <- quantile(subTI$Tail.intensity, 0.9)
> succ <- tapply(TIComet$Tail.intensity, TIComet$Animal_no,
+                 function(x) sum(x > cutpoint))
> fail <- tapply(TIComet$Tail.intensity, TIComet$Animal_no,
+                 function(x) sum(x <= cutpoint))
```

Table 4.17: 90th Percentile Dichotomized Data

Responder	Nonresponder	Treatment	Animal No.
5	95	VC	1
10	90	VC	2
15	85	VC	3
9	91	VC	4
11	89	VC	5
7	93	Low	6
18	82	Low	7
12	88	Low	8
13	87	Low	9
28	72	Low	10
35	65	medium	11
54	46	medium	12
71	29	medium	13
70	30	medium	14
51	49	medium	15
70	30	High	16
54	46	High	17
55	45	High	18
77	23	High	19
64	36	High	20
80	20	Superhigh	21
73	27	Superhigh	22
75	25	Superhigh	23
71	29	Superhigh	24
82	18	Superhigh	25

```
> TIresp <-TIrespond[, c(1,2,5)]
> TII <-table( TIresp$Dose, TIresp$responder)
> mosaicplot(TII, main="", color=TRUE)
> library("multcomp")
> library("lme4")
> TIrespond$Dose <-factor(TIrespond$Treatment,
+                    levels(TIrespond$Treatment)[c(5,2,3,1,4)])
> modTI1 <- glmer(cbind(succ, fail) ~ Dose-1 + (1|Animal_no),
+                 data=TIrespond, family=binomial(link="logit"))
> plot(glht(modTI1, linfct = mcp(Dose = "Dunnett"), alternative="greater"),
+      main="", xlab=" ")
```

Figure 4.13a shows the number of responders, i.e., the number of values above the 90th
percentile of control, where a clear dose-related pattern can be seen. The related Dunnett-

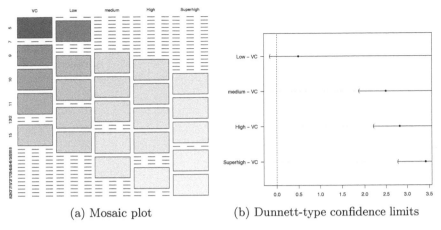

(a) Mosaic plot   (b) Dunnett-type confidence limits

FIGURE 4.13: 90th percentile responder rates.

type one-sided lower confidence limits for these overdispersed proportions, modeled by a generalized mixed-effects model, are shown in Figure 4.13b. A clear dose-related increasing effect can be seen above the low dose.

Second, the simple approach using log-transformed tail intensities is used (see the boxplots in Figure 4.14a). However, the effect size of expected median differences ([338]) should be interpreted correctly and the finite properties of simultaneous inference in the mixed model, additionally with variance heterogeneity is unknown. The lower confidence limits for Dunnett-type inference in Figure 4.14b show again a strong dose-related effect.

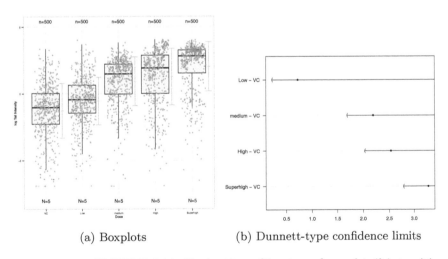

(a) Boxplots   (b) Dunnett-type confidence limits

FIGURE 4.14: Evaluation of log-transformed tail intensities.

The next two approaches assume a bimodal mixing distribution of two normally distributed variables: responder and non-responder. Here, the responder category is estimated by model based-clustering using the R package `flexmix` [134], not just by a naive percentile rule. Assuming certain prior probabilities for being a responder (or not) on an animal level, a mixture of two linear models can be fitted with the animal number as a factor. The resulting posterior probabilities are obtained for a partitioning into the two clusters: responder and non-responder. Figure 4.15a shows the related mosaic plot. These proportions are analyzed by Dunnett-type inference, where the between-animal variability is modeled assuming overdispersed proportions in the generalized linear model (third approach). Notice, the confidence limits in Figure 4.15b are on the logit link, i.e., the value of $H_0 = 1$. A back-transformation on the odds ratio scale is possible.

```
> library("toxbox")
> library("flexmix")
> leisch <- flexmix(Tail.intensity ~ 1, data = TIComet,
+                    k=2, control=list(minprior=0))
> cf <- clusters(leisch)
> TIComet$fcat <- as.integer(cf-1)
> mosaicplot(Treatment~fcat, data=TIComet, main="", color=TRUE)
> Lmod2 <- glm(fcat ~ Treatment, data=TIComet,
+              family=quasibinomial(link="logit"))
> plot(glht(Lmod2, linfct = mcp(Treatment = "Dunnett"),
+           alternative="greater"),
+ main="", xlab="Simultaneous confidence interval on logit link scale")
```

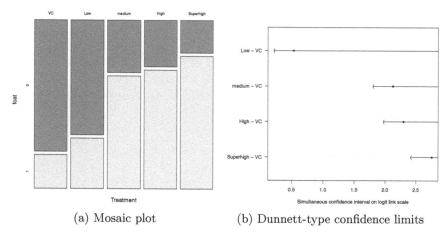

(a) Mosaic plot   (b) Dunnett-type confidence limits

FIGURE 4.15: Evaluation of bimodal distributed responder rates.

The fourth approach selects the responder values only (see the seriously unbalanced design in the boxplots in Figure 4.16a) and estimated Dunnett-type limits using a mixed model; see Figure 4.16b. (Notice, group 1 in the object `fcat==1` is not necessarily the responder in any dataset due to the specific program style of `flexmix`.)

```
> library("toxbox")
> boxclust(data=subset(TIComet, fcat==1), outcome="Tail.intensity",
+          treatment="Treatment", cluster="Animal_no",
+          ylabel="Tail Intensity of responder only", xlabel="Dose",
+          option="dotplot", psize=1.5, hjitter=0.1, legpos="none",
+          printN="TRUE", white=TRUE, titlesize=8, labelsize=6)
> library("lme4")
> mmLH <- lmer(Tail.intensity ~ Treatment-1 + (1|Treatment:Animal_no)
+              + (1|Treatment:Animal_no:Sample),
+              data=subset(TIComet, fcat==1))
```

```
> plot(glht(mmLH, linfct=mcp(Treatment="Dunnett"), alternative="greater"),
+           main="", xlab=" ")
```

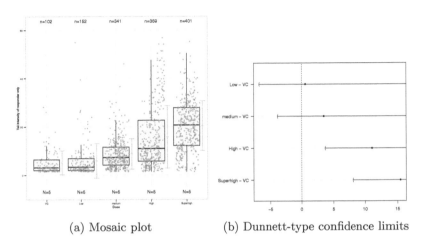

(a) Mosaic plot   (b) Dunnett-type confidence limits

FIGURE 4.16: Evaluating responding animals only.

Of course, one cannot say which is the most appropriate method, and certainly not on the basis of the data. For this purpose, extensive simulation studies and the comparative analysis of several assays are needed. Differently to a proposed simplified analysis using median of all sub-units within an animal as endpoint data [247, 57], all four approaches model the between animal (sample) variability. A nonparametric version would be appropriate for such skewed data (see Section 2.1.4), but such an approach is not available in a mixed effects framework.

4.13 Evaluation of the *in vitro* micronucleus assay as an example for comparing cell distributions

In the *in vitro* micronucleus assay among others the distribution of mono-, bi-, tri- and tetra-nucleated cells should be considered according to the related guideline [290]. Therefore, the problem of comparing cell distribution functions (instead of a single endpoint) arises [125]. As an example the number of cells carrying one, two, and three micronuclei after the exposure to X-ray radiation [156] (in their Table 2) is used.

```
> data("he", package="SiTuR")
> hes <- he[,-8]
```

In these data, three problems are visible in Table 4.18: i) between-donor variability (even two donors only), ii) non-zero information for the category *three micronuclei*, and iii) zero counts in the doses 0.02, 0.05, and 0.10 for the pathological relevant *two or three micronuclei*

Table 4.18: Mono-, Bi- and Tri-Nucleated Cell Counts

group	donor	NC	one	two	three	total
control	a	1000	8	0	0	8
d0.02	a	1000	10	0	0	10
d0.05	a	1000	16	0	0	16
d0.10	a	1000	14	0	0	14
d0.25	a	1000	23	1	0	24
d0.50	a	1000	24	2	0	26
d1.00	a	1000	36	5	0	41
d2.00	a	1000	53	7	2	62
control	b	1000	7	0	0	7
d0.02	b	1000	8	0	0	8
d0.05	b	1000	7	0	0	7
d0.10	b	1000	9	0	0	9
d0.25	b	1000	11	0	0	11
d0.50	b	1000	16	1	0	17
d1.00	b	1000	24	2	0	26
d2.00	b	1000	56	4	1	61

categories. By pooling over donors, defining the category `two+` and eliminating the low doses, a simplified 5-by-3 table results in Table 4.19:

Table 4.19: No, Mono-, Bi-Nucleated Cell Counts Pooled over Donors

no	one	two+
1985	15	0
1965	34	1
1957	40	3
1933	60	7
1877	109	14

These counts can be assumed to follow a multinomial distribution, as the complete number of scored cells (NC) is known. The evaluation of multinomial models using the package `mmcp` is described in Section 2.1.7 in detail.

The R function `multinomMCP` in the package `mmcp` [127] constructs a joint contrast matrix, matching the parameterization of the multinomial model, by setting up two contrasts, one for category comparisons and the other for any factor level comparisons. If only categories are compared on one specific factor level, the parameter of interest can be interpreted in terms of an odds ratio as the proportion of counts in one category divided by the proportion of counts in the baseline category (i.e., non-nucleated), for example, performing a Dunnett contrast for dose groups and a Dunnett-type for categories against non-nucleated cells. Because of the zero cell counts, the odds ratios are large and the confidence intervals unstable. The object `mmcpt` contains eight adjusted p-values for i) the comparison of each dose against control and ii) for the comparison of the categories one and two+ against non-nucleated cells. All comparisons larger than 0.25 mg/kg are highly significant.

```
> library("mmcp")
> mmcpT <- multinomMCP(Counts, Fac, groups = "Dunnett", endp = "Dunnett",
+                        char.length=5)
> mmcpt <-summary(mmcpT)
```

Notice, this approach allows a c-by-k table data structure only, e.g., overdispersion is not considered. For a general approach to compare cell distribution further work is needed.

5

Evaluation of reproductive toxicity assays

5.1 The statistical problems

The appropriate statistical evaluation of reproduction/development studies, particularly multi-generation assays [200], is rather complex. The most important feature of reproductive assays is the correlation between the litter mates within a dam. The simpler teratogenicity study will be used here for demonstration purposes, where pregnant females are treated with the test compound in a randomized design including several dose groups and a negative control. At a certain stage of gestation the females are sacrified and several reproductive parameters such as number of pre-implantations, implantations, alive or dead pups, malformations, and pup weights are estimated for each pup within each female. Statistically two major problems exist: i) modeling the sub-unit *litter mates* within the randomized experimental unit *female*, so-called per-litter analysis (recommended by the ICH-guideline [200]) and, ii) modeling the possible competition between early loss/mortality and malformation of the pups. The first problem is split methodologically into a mixed model for the continuous endpoint pup weight and into a mixed model for correlated proportions for the incidence endpoints. The second problem is even more complex and will be discussed only briefly in Sections 5.3.2 and 5.4. Finally, female-specific endpoints occur also, such as number of corpora lutea. Their analysis can be easily performed by nonparametric Dunnett/Williams-type procedure (see Section 1.2.6)

Features:

- Per-litter analysis for continuous endpoints, such as pup weight

- Per-litter analysis for proportions, such as malformation rate

- Analysis of different-scaled multiple endpoints, such as pup weight and malformation rate

- Analysis of female-specific endpoints, such as corpora lutea

- Analysis of behavioral data

5.2   Evaluation of the continuous endpoint pup weight

A dose-related weight reduction of the pups within the litters can be interpreted as a terato-
genic effect. A Williams-type trend test in the mixed model with either adjusted p-values
or simultaneous confidence intervals will be used. Instead of using the common linear model
estimates, a mixed model containing both fixed effects (*dose*) and random effects (*litter*)
is appropriate. It is the preferred approach for modeling correlated continuous data, such
as repeated measures, technical replicates, paired organs, and within-litter dependencies
[305, 391]. As a data example we use a textbook example [390] where in a randomized
design 30 female rats were randomly assigned to receive control, low, or high dose of an
experimental compound.

```
> data("ratpup", package="WWGbook")
> Ratpup <-ratpup
> Ratpup$Treatment <-factor(Ratpup$treatment,
+                   levels=c("Control","Low","High"))
> Ratpup$adjLitsize <- Ratpup$litsize- mean(Ratpup$litsize)
```

In total, 322 observations are available for the following 6 variables: *pup.id, weight, sex,
litter (litter ID), litsize (litter size) and treatment*; see Table 5.1. Already this data structure makes the specificity clear: the data do not contain just the endpoint pup weight and
the treatment levels like in most chronic, carcinogenicity, and mutagenicity assays; it also
contains an identifier for the particular litter. Importantly, because of the potential relationship between litter size and litter weight, the data also contain the subsequently used
covariate *litter size*.

Already the three boxplots in Figure 5.1 make the differences between the statistical approaches clear: i) assuming the pup as experimental unit, i.e., per-fetus analysis (*left panel*),
ii) assuming pups as sub-units within the randomized unit litter, i.e., per-litter analysis
(*middle panel*), and iii) mean pup weight per litter (*right panel*), i.e., simplified analysis.

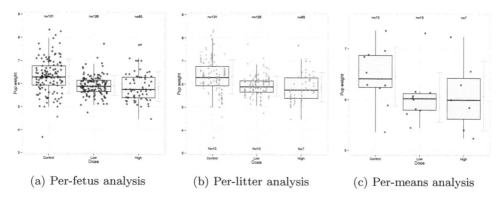

(a) Per-fetus analysis   (b) Per-litter analysis   (c) Per-means analysis

FIGURE 5.1: Boxplots for three data models.

The differences are obvious: the per-fetus analysis (*left*) uses virtually large sample sizes,
the mean value consideration (*right*) ignores the different litter sizes, whereas the per-

Table 5.1: Pup Weight Data

pup.id	weight	sex	litter	litsize	treatment
1	6.60	Male	1	12	Control
2	7.40	Male	1	12	Control
3	7.15	Male	1	12	Control
4	7.24	Male	1	12	Control
5	7.10	Male	1	12	Control
6	6.04	Male	1	12	Control
7	6.98	Male	1	12	Control
8	7.05	Male	1	12	Control
9	6.95	Female	1	12	Control
10	6.29	Female	1	12	Control
11	6.77	Female	1	12	Control
12	6.57	Female	1	12	Control
13	6.37	Male	2	14	Control
14	6.37	Male	2	14	Control
15	6.90	Male	2	14	Control
...	...	...	...	...	...
311	6.42	Female	26	9	High
312	6.42	Female	26	9	High
313	6.30	Female	26	9	High
314	5.64	Male	27	9	High
315	6.08	Male	27	9	High
316	6.56	Male	27	9	High
317	6.29	Male	27	9	High
318	5.69	Male	27	9	High
319	6.36	Male	27	9	High
320	5.93	Female	27	9	High
321	5.74	Female	27	9	High
322	5.74	Female	27	9	High

litter analysis (*middle*) is the appropriate approach. (Notice, package `toxbox` contains a `color=TRUE` option, which makes the differences between the models clearer.) A mixed effects model can be used with *treatment* as fixed factor and *litter* as random factor [421]:

```
> library("nlme")
> mix1 <- lme(weight ~ Treatment, random=~1|litter, data=Ratpup)
> library("multcomp")
> mixaa <-summary(glht(mix1, linfct = mcp(Treatment = "Dunnett"),
+               alternative="less"))
> pvalmix <-round(mixaa$test$pvalues, 3)
> naivm <- lm(weight ~ Treatment, data=Ratpup)
> pvalnaiv <-summary(glht(naivm, linfct = mcp(Treatment = "Dunnett"),
+               alternative="less"))$test$pvalues
```

The adjusted *p*-value for the one-sided Dunnett-type comparison high dose against control for the mixed effects model (using *treatment* as fixed factor and *litter* as random factor) is 0.125 (in the object `pvalmix`), compared with naive (and inappropriately liberal) model taking all pups as pseudo-experimental units with of *p*-value of 4×10^{-6} (per-fetus analysis). Simply, in this naive approach the sample sizes in the control group n=131, n=126, n=65 are much larger than the randomized samples sizes of N=10, N=10, N=7.

```
> mix2 <- lme(weight ~ Treatment+sex+adjLitsize, random=~1|litter,
+         data=Ratpup, weights = varIdent(form = ~1 | Treatment))
> pvalcompl <-summary(glht(mix2, linfct = mcp(Treatment = "Dunnett"),
```

+   `alternative="less"))$test$pvalues`

The question arises whether this simple mixed model taking only the factor `treatment` into account is appropriate whereas a secondary factor `sex` and a covariate `adjLitsize` (i.e., the litter size as difference to its total mean) exist. Moreover, the variance heterogeneity in the unbalanced design (see Figure 5.1) should be considered. Two strategies exist: to take the complete model or to compare different models and selected the sparest one. The above selected detailed mixed model reveals a strong weight reduction effect: the *p*-value for high dose against control is 2×10^{-6} (instead of 0.125 in the simple mixed model without considering the covariate litter size!) which is mainly caused by the strong group-specific relationship between weight and litter size [76]. Commonly the litter size should be included as a covariate for continuous endpoints such as pup weight [72]. Even more complex models can be established by considering interactions or Bayesian approaches for joint analysis of pup weight and litter size by a shared latent variable model [103] or its extension to correlated random effects [136, 137]. Notice, the use of the covariate `adjLitsize` requires several assumptions, which may be violated; in the example the covariate `litsize` itself depends monotonically on `dose`; see Figure 5.2. For further details on the assumptions for a covariate see Section 2.4.4 or the recent summary paper [207].

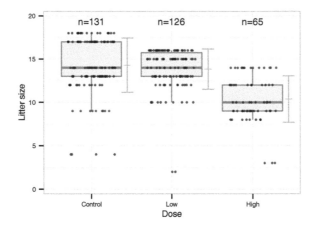

FIGURE 5.2: Boxplots for the covariate litter size as endpoint.

5.2.1 Possible simplification?

The correct unbiased use of a mixed effect model with a possibly treatment-dependent covariate for small sample size designs may be a challenge. Therefore, the question arise whether a simplified evaluation using just the litter means as a pseudo-endpoint can be an alternative; see the related boxplots in the right panel of Figure 5.1. Notice, only in a balanced one-way layout with a primary fixed factor (dose) and a secondary random variable (litter), the means over the secondary factors are unbiased estimates. Already unbalancedness introduces a bias, typically in teratogenicity studies per definition:

Table 5.2: Summary Statistics (Mean, Standard Deviation): Per-Fetus vs. Litter Mean Data

	Per-fetus			Mean-litter data		
Control	6.325	0.745	n=131	6.467	0.579	n=10
Low	5.928	0.427	n=126	6.054	0.494	n=10
High	5.886	0.644	n=65	6.085	0.687	n=7

```
> library("multcomp")
> Mnaiv <- lm(Meanweight ~ Treatment+Litsize, data=litM)
> pvalnaivM <-summary(glht(Mnaiv, linfct = mcp(Treatment = "Dunnett"),
+                          alternative="less"))$test$pvalues
```

We see already from Table 5.2 that the means over all pup weights are different compared with the means over the litter means (as well as standard deviations and sample sizes). Therefore the *p*-value of 0.0023 for comparing the high dose against control for this simplified approach differs also from that of mixed model approach. The more the litter sizes differ, the more biased is the simplified approach. Therefore, such a simplification cannot be recommended for routine analysis.

5.3 Evaluation of proportions

Most of the relevant endpoints in reprotoxicity studies are proportions, such as number of malformations, implantations, or dead fetuses relative to the number of pups. These proportions are estimated per litter, and therefore an extra-binomial variation, i.e., between litters within a treatment group, occurs. A naive analysis by 2-by-k table data, i.e., just the single summarized proportions per treatment groups, ignores this between-litter variability, and cannot be recommended. Several approaches for modeling extra-binomial variability are available, among them a mixed-effects model approach similar to the analysis of continuous data (see Section 2.1.5.4.1). Here we focus on a quasi-binomial link-function `family=quasibinomial(link="logit")` in the generalized linear model, a seemingly robust approach.

As a data example, the iron-deficient diet study with a control and three iron supplement schedules is used (available in the `library(VGAM)` [268]).

```
> data("lirat", package="VGAM")
> lirat$ID <- as.factor(1:nrow(lirat))
> lirat$treatment <-as.factor(lirat$grp)
> lirat$Prop <-lirat$R/lirat$N+0.00001
```

As endpoint the number of dead fetuses (R) per number of fetuses within a female rat (N) is considered; see the raw data in Table 5.3. This study is more pharmacologically instead of toxicologically oriented and the question should be answered, which supplement schedule causes the smallest proportion of dead fetuses versus control, i.e., a one-sided Dunnett-type procedure for a decrease is used. For each litter the number of dead fetuses is considered to be binomial (N,p) distributed where p varies from litter to litter. The total variance of the proportions will be greater because of the between-litter variability. The common variance $var() = p_i(1-p_i)$ is extended by inclusion of a dispersion parameter $\tau > 1$ $var() = \tau p_i(1-p_i)$, called overdispersion. Therefore we use the generalized linear model with quasibinomial link function to estimate the dispersion parameter.

Table 5.3: Proportion of Dead Fetuses—Raw Data

N	R	ID	treatment	Prop
10	1	1	1	0.10
11	4	2	1	0.36
12	9	3	1	0.75
4	4	4	1	1.00
10	10	5	1	1.00
11	9	6	1	0.82

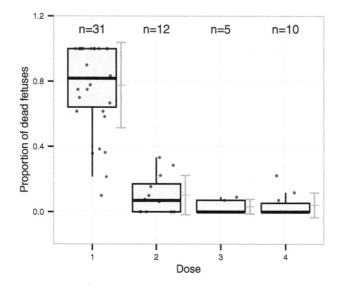

FIGURE 5.3: Boxplots for the proportions of dead fetuses.

```
> library("multcomp")
> mp1 <- glm(cbind(R, N-R) ~ treatment-1, data=lirat,
+            family=quasibinomial(link="logit"))
> disp<-round(summary(mp1)$dispersion,2)
> gg <- glht(mp1, linfct = mcp(treatment = "Dunnett"),
+            alternative="less")
> gg$df <- df.residual(mp1)
> pValues<-summary(gg)
> deadF<-exp(confint(gg)$confint)[,-2]
```

For each female within a treatment group the proportion of dead pups was estimated. The boxplots in Figure 5.3 show the many extreme proportions of 1 or 0, the decreasing effect for any supplementary diet, and much larger variance in the control. Within the general-

Table 5.4: Dunnett-Type Analysis of Proportion of Dead Fetuses Taking Overdispersion into Account

	Odds ratio	Upper confidence limit
2 - 1	0.036	0.122
3 - 1	0.011	0.167
4 - 1	0.016	0.093

ized linear model the link function `quasibinomial(link="logit")` was used allowing the estimation of a dispersion parameter. In the example a dispersion parameter of 2.86 was estimated, i.e., a substantial overdispersion exists. The *p*-values for the one-sided Dunnett procedures indicate for any diet a strong significant decrease of the death rate versus the iron-deficit in the control. Because of using the logit link function, odds ratios are the point estimators, i.e., the k-fold of a chance for a litter to have a smaller dead rate than the control. Table 5.4 shows the odds ratios and their upper confidence limit; upper, because we are interested in the pharmacological effect of reducing the number of dead fetuses. In the boxplots we see an extreme variance heterogeneity, possibly treatment-dependent. Therefore, a related adjusted Dunnett-type procedure is suggested [147]) and is used here in combination with the sandwich estimator to account for the variance heterogeneity [159]. Alternatively, tests for group-specific overdispersion are available [334, 333] to account for variance heterogeneity.

```
> library("sandwich")
> gS <- glht(mp1, linfct = mcp(treatment = "Dunnett"),
+            alternative="less", vcov=vcovHC)
> gS$df <- df.residual(mp1)
> pValueS<-summary(gS)
> deadSW<-exp(confint(gS)$confint)[,-2]
```

Table 5.5: Dunnett-Type Analysis of Proportion of Dead Fetuses Adjusted for Variance Heterogeneity

	Odds ratio	Upper confidence limit
2 - 1	0.036	0.101
3 - 1	0.011	0.057
4 - 1	0.016	0.065

In Table 5.5 the smallest upper confidence limit belongs to group 3 (injections on days 0 and 7; see [268]); quite differently to the analysis assuming homogeneous variances in Table 5.4.

Alternatively, a mixed model can be used where the litter (ID) is used a random factor –analogously to the evaluation of continuous endpoints in Section 5.2. Further approaches are available, such as using a betabinomial model (e.g., by the `library(VGAM)` [410], or the generalized estimation equation approach for correlated binomial endpoints [292] (e.g., by packages **gee, geepack**. The advantage of GEE-methods is that the distribution of the endpoint must be exactly specified and they provide a robust estimate of the variance even when the working correlation matrix is mis-specified and missings (completely at random) occur. A Dunnett-type GEE approach was proposed a decade ago [292] but the computation of either adjusted p-values or simultaneous confidence limits was difficult. Surprisingly, no follow-up papers exist. By means of the packages `geepack, multcomp` both adjusted p-values and confidence limits can be estimated for any multiple contrast, such as Dunnett- or Williams-type. The function `geeglm` allows a GLM-style model specification, such as `family=binomial`, and the definition of the correlation structure `corstr=exchangeable` for clustered-binomial data. As data example, the litter-specific number of abnormal pups in a common design was used [298].

```
> data("paul", package="SiTuR")
```

In Table 5.6 we see the data structure with `Treatment, Litter, Abnormal` and serious between litter heterogeneities of the abnormal rate.

Table 5.6: Raw Data of Litter-Specific Abnormal Pup Counts

Treatment	Litter	Abnormal
Control	1	0
Control	1	0
Control	1	0
Control	1	0
Control	1	0
Control	1	0
Control	1	0
Control	1	0
Control	1	0
Control	1	0
Control	1	0
...	...	...
High	78	0
High	78	1
High	78	1
High	79	0
High	79	0
High	79	0
High	79	0
High	79	0
High	79	1
High	79	1
High	79	1
High	80	0
High	80	0
High	80	0
High	80	0
High	80	0
High	80	1

Using the packages `geepack` and `multcomp` a Dunnett- or Williams-type test can be easily performed.

The mosaic plot in Figure 5.4a provides a crude overview about the abnormal rate without considering the quite different litter sizes.

```
> library("geepack")
> library("multcomp")
> paul$treat<-factor(paul$Treatment,
```

```
+                 levels=c("Control","Low","Medium", "High"))
> mosaicplot(treat~Abnormal, data=paul, main="", color=TRUE)
> paulgee <- geeglm(Abnormal ~ treat-1, data=paul, id=Litter,
+                 family=binomial, corstr="exch")
> mycontrmat <- rbind("C3" = c(-1, 0, 0, 1),
+                 "C2" = c(-1, 0, 1/2, 1/2),
+                 "C1" = c(-1, 1/3,1/3,1/3),
+                 "C-H" = c(-1, 0,0,1),
+                 "C-M" = c(-1, 0,1,0),
+                 "C-L" = c(-1, 1,0,0))
> paulDU<-glht(parm(coef=coef(paulgee), vcov=paulgee$geese$vbeta),
+                 linfct=mycontrmat, alternative="greater")
> plot(paulDU, main="", xlab="Simultaneous confidence interval")
```

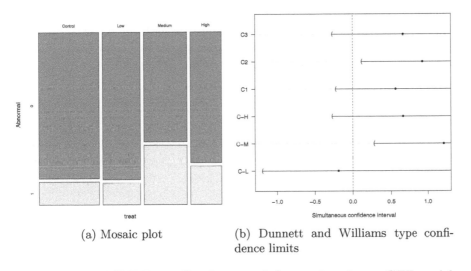

(a) Mosaic plot   (b) Dunnett and Williams type confidence limits

FIGURE 5.4: Simultaneous inference based on a GEE model.

From the lower simultaneous confidence limits in Figure 5.4b we see a substantial increase of the abnormal rate in the medium dose (and in the Williams-contrast C2, which represents pooled high and mid dose). Unfortunately, this simple and robust approach cannot be recommended today because detailed comparisons between the three main approaches (GEE, mixed-effects model, generalized linear model with overdispersed proportions) are not available up to now.

5.3.1   Possible simplification?

Instead of using the previous generalized linear model approach, a simple transformations of proportions into a pseudo-normal endpoint can be used under some conditions, such as the arcsine transformation [135] proposed by the US NTP [9] and discussed in detail in Section 2.1.5.4.3. Two disadvantages occur: the effect size and its confidence interval for such a transformed endpoint cannot really be interpreted (i.e., only p-values can be used), and the transformation properties are commonly acceptable only for large sample sizes. On the other hand, transformations are simple to use:

```
> lirat$Prop<-lirat$R/lirat$N
> lirat$AS<-asin(sqrt(lirat$Prop))
> mas<-lm(AS~treatment, data=lirat)
> library("sandwich")
> sp<-summary(glht(mas, linfct=mcp(treatment = "Dunnett"),
+                  vcov=vcovHC, alternative="less"))
```

Using the sandwich estimator for the covariance matrix allows heterogeneous variances in the treatment groups. The resulting Dunnett-type p-values (in the object sp) are much smaller than the above direct approach taking the overdispersion of proportions into account. Alternatively the rank-based Dunnett test can be used for the female-specific proportions.

```
> lirat$Prop<-lirat$R/lirat$N
> library("nparcomp")
> rp<-summary(nparcomp(Prop ~treatment, data=lirat, asy.method = "mult.t",
+                type = "Dunnett", alternative = "less", info = FALSE))
```

Again, much smaller p-values (in the object rp) result compared with the direct approach. As long as systematic simulation studies comparing the direct with the simplified methods are missing, these simplified methods cannot be recommended for the routine.

5.3.2   Analysis of multiple binary findings

Multiple binary data occur frequently in toxicology, e.g., multiple tumors in long-term carcinogenicity studies (see Section 3.6.1) and multiple findings in reproductive toxicity studies. Commonly, these proportions are analyzed independently, each at level α. Some approaches for jointly analyzing multiple binary data exist; see Section 2.1.5.5. As a data example the two binary endpoints: variations and malformations in a reproductive study on diethylene glycol dimethyl ether [8] are available on pup level (without dose group $62.5mg/kg$ to avoid the zero-proportion problem).

```
> # per-foetus level
> data("bivar", package="SiTuR")
> bivar1 <- bivar
> bivar1$Malformation <- ifelse(bivar1$DEFECT_TYPE=="Malformation", 1, 0)
> bivar1$Variation <- ifelse(bivar1$DEFECT_TYPE=="Variation", 1, 0)
> bivar1$None <- ifelse(bivar1$DEFECT_TYPE=="", 1, 0)
> bivar1$dose <- as.factor(bivar1$DOSE)
> bivar1$dam <- as.factor(bivar1$DAM_ID)
> bivarE<-bivar1[bivar1$dose!="62.5", ]
> bivarX<-bivarE[, c(4:8)]
```

The correlation between the two binary endpoints Malformations and Variations is rather specific, depending on the fetus or litter level. Thus, a per-fetus and per-litter analysis is discussed here.

The data on pup level are given in Table 5.7. Up to now, only a per-fetus analysis can be used, assuming incorrectly the pup as experimental unit, i.e., the sample sizes are virtually large. First for each endpoint a marginal generalized linear model is fitted (m1, m2), where the odds ratio is the effect size using the logit link. Second the joint distribution of both endpoints modeled using the function mmm in the R package multcomp.

Table 5.7: Malformations and Variations on Pup Level Raw Data

Malformation	Variation	None	dose	dam
0	0	1	0	51
0	0	1	0	51
0	0	1	0	51
0	0	1	0	51
0	0	1	0	51
0	0	1	0	51
0	0	1	0	51
0	0	1	0	51
0	0	1	0	51
0	0	1	0	51
...	...	...	...	...
0	0	1	500	185
0	0	1	500	185
0	0	1	500	185
0	0	1	500	185
0	0	1	500	185
1	0	0	500	185
0	1	0	500	185
0	1	0	500	185
0	0	1	500	185

```
> m1<-glm(cbind(Malformation,None)~dose, data=bivarE,
+           family = binomial(), na.action="na.exclude")
> m2<-glm(cbind(Variation,None)~dose, data=bivarE,
+           family = binomial(), na.action="na.exclude")
> library("multcomp")
> m12 <- glht(mmm(Mal = m1, Var= m2),  mlf(mcp(dose ="Dunnett")),
+               alternative="greater")
```

Table 5.8: Per-Fetus Analysis of Variations and Malformations Jointly

	Estimate	p-value
1	Mal: 125 - 0	0.1153
2	Mal: 250 - 0	0.0000
3	Mal: 500 - 0	0.0000
4	Var: 125 - 0	0.0004
5	Var: 250 - 0	0.0000
6	Var: 500 - 0	0.0000

Table 5.8 shows the multiplicity-adjusted p-values for both malformations (Mal) and variations (Var) for all many-to-one comparisons. Strong increases of both malformations and variations occur in almost any doses (except in the low dose for variations). However, these tiny p-values are not surprising because of the pseudo-large sample sizes.

A second per-fetus style of analysis assumes for the multiple binary endpoints a multinomial vector. A data example was selected with three binary endpoints, namely the developmental toxicity of diethylene glycol dimethyl ether in mice [312]; see Table 5.9 and in Figure 5.5 the related mosaic plot.

```
> kimmel<-data.frame(
+ dose = c(0,62.5, 125, 250, 500),
+ alive = c(281, 225,283,202,9),
+ dead = c(15, 17, 22, 38, 144),
+ malformed = c(1, 0, 7, 59, 132))
> library("xtable")
> kimTAB<-xtable(kimmel, digits=c(0,1,0,0,0),
+                 caption="Per-fetus Table Data of Dead,
+                 Malformed, and Surviving Pups", label="tab:kimmel")
> print(kimTAB, table.placement = "H", caption.placement = "top")

> mtox<-as.matrix(kimmel[,2:4])
> rownames(mtox)<-kimmel[,1]
> mosaicplot(mtox,  las=2, main="", color=TRUE)
```

Table 5.9: Per-Fetus Table Data of Dead, Malformed, and Surviving Pups

	dose	alive	dead	malformed
1	0.0	281	15	1
2	62.5	225	17	0
3	125.0	283	22	7
4	250.0	202	38	59
5	500.0	9	144	132

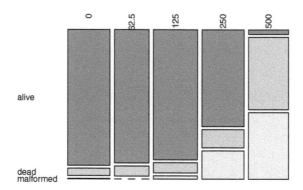

FIGURE 5.5: Mosaic plot for dead, malformed and surviving pups.

Using the function `multnomMCP` the log odds ratio for comparisons of the doses against control and of the pathological categories against alive can be estimated, together with their simultaneous confidence limits.

```
> library("nnet")
> library("mmcp")
> ctox <- as.matrix(cbind(mtox[,c(1:3)]+1))# add1
> colnames(ctox) <- c("alive", "dead","malformed")
> multox <- multinomMCP(ctox, as.factor(kimmel$dose),
+             groups = "Dunnett", endp ="Dunnett", char.length=10,
+             trace=FALSE)
```

```
> multoxp <- summary(multox)
```

In the object `multoxp` the multiplicity-adjusted p-values for the log odds ratios for Dunnett-type dose vs. control comparisons and categories vs. alive comparisons. For both 500 and 250 dose group significantly increasing odds ratios for both dead/alive and malformed/alive exist. A third approach is based on a per-litter data structure which can be achieved when cumulating the findings for each litter; see Table 5.10 for the diethylene glycol dimethyl ether data.

Table 5.10: Malformations and Variations on Litter Level Data

Malformations	Variations	None	Total	dose
0	0	10	10	0
0	0	14	14	0
0	1	11	12	0
0	0	17	17	0
0	0	15	15	0
0	0	17	17	0
2	1	11	14	0
...	...	...	...	...
7	4	11	22	500
35	22	5	62	500
8	11	9	28	500
18	7	6	31	500
37	21	7	65	500
2	2	9	13	500

Again, for each proportion a marginal generalized linear model is fitted (`mL1`, `mL2`) but now a quasibinomial link is used to account for overdispersion between the litter.

```
> library("multcomp")
> mL1<-glm(cbind(Malformations,None)~dose, data=bivarY,
+          family = quasibinomial(), na.action="na.exclude")
> mL2<-glm(cbind(Variations,None)~dose, data=bivarY,
+          family = quasibinomial(), na.action="na.exclude")
> mL12 <- glht(mmm(Mal = mL1, Var= mL2),  mlf(mcp(dose ="Dunnett")),
+              alternative="greater")
```

Table 5.11: Per-Litter Analysis of Variations and Malformations Jointly

Comparison	Test statistics	p-value
Mal: 125 - 0	1.05	0.373305
Mal: 250 - 0	3.09	0.003938
Mal: 500 - 0	4.89	0.000002
Var: 125 - 0	2.39	0.031110
Var: 250 - 0	2.88	0.008199
Var: 500 - 0	6.75	0.000000

Now, the multiplicity-adjusted p-values in Table 5.11 are larger than those for the per-fetus analysis because of modeling the overdispersion. In the objects `mL1`, `mL2` substantial overdispersion can be seen. Now malformations and variations reveal an increase against control for the medium and high dose only.

5.4 Analysis of different-scaled multiple endpoints

The dependencies between differently scaled multiple endpoints, such as pup weight, fetal death and malformation rate, and the covariate dose can be analyzed by specific regression models [73], weighted for potential outcomes using principal strata [107], threshold models [114], or bivariate random effects models [274, 244]. Moreover, benchmark dose models for per-litter data are available [25] for which a threshold dose-response model with random litter effects [196] was proposed. As an example the ethylene glycol data from a developmental toxicity study conducted by the National Toxicology Program [312] are available [408].

```
> data("wuleon", package="SiTuR")
```

Ninety four pregnant mice were randomly exposed to ethyl glycol at four different dose levels, 0, 0.75, 1.5, and 3 g/kg/day (with dose 0 as control), and 1028 live fetuses (with litter sizes ranging from 1 to 16) were examined for various defects, including fetal weight (continuous) and the presence/absence of fetal malformations (binary), both believed to be sensitive indicators of toxicity. Figure 5.6 shows the pup weights and the malformation rates on a per-fetus level; see the raw data in Table 5.12.

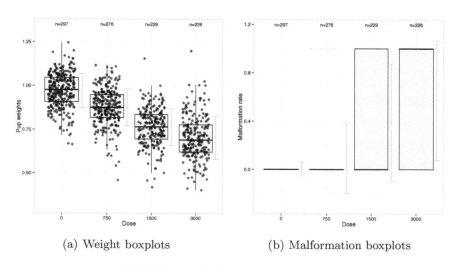

(a) Weight boxplots   (b) Malformation boxplots

FIGURE 5.6: Ethylen glycol example.

An alternative to trend tests considering the qualitative factor `dose`, trend tests were proposed for the qualitative covariate `Dose`. Here we use a modification of the maximum test on three regression models for the arithmetic, ordinal, and logarithmic-linear dose metameters

Table 5.12: Raw Data of Fetal Weights and Malformations

Litter	Dose	Weight	Malformation
60	0	0.90	0
60	0	0.83	0
60	0	0.95	0
60	0	0.95	0
60	0	1.07	0
60	0	1.06	0
60	0	0.96	0
61	0	1.02	0
61	0	1.01	0
61	0	1.07	0
61	0	0.82	0
61	0	1.01	0
61	0	0.99	0
61	0	1.06	0
61	0	1.04	0
61	0	1.02	0
61	0	1.04	0
61	0	0.91	0
...	...	...	...
156	3000	0.79	0
156	3000	0.90	0
156	3000	0.86	0
156	3000	0.86	0
156	3000	0.80	0
156	3000	0.84	0
156	3000	0.87	0
156	3000	0.72	0
156	3000	0.83	0

[380]. Using the concept of multiple marginal models [307] allows not only to obtain the joint distribution of these three slope parameters without assuming a certain multivariate distribution for the data, but also the simultaneous evaluation of possibly different-scaled multiple endpoints via inclusion of multiple marginal generalized linear models into the related function mmm within the R package multcomp [189, 190]. In the above ethylene glycol example the three objects wN, wO, wLL contain the parameter estimates of linear models for the normal distributed endpoint Weight and further the three objects pN, pO, pLL containing the parameter estimates of generalized linear models with binomial link functions for the binary endpoint Malformation.

```
> library("multcomp")
> wuleon$dose<-as.factor(wuleon$Dose)
> Dlevelw<-as.numeric(levels(wuleon$dose))
> SOW<-log(Dlevelw[2])-
+    log(Dlevelw[3]/Dlevelw[2])*(Dlevelw[2]-Dlevelw[1])/(Dlevelw[3]-Dlevelw[2])
> wuleon$DoseN<-as.numeric(as.character(wuleon$dose))
> wuleon$DoseO<-as.numeric(wuleon$dose)
> wuleon$DoseL<-log(wuleon$DoseN)
> wuleon$DoseLL<-wuleon$DoseL
> wuleon$DoseLL[wuleon$DoseN==Dlevelw[1]] <-SOW
>
> wN <-lm(Weight~DoseN, data=wuleon)
> wO <-lm(Weight~DoseO, data=wuleon)
```

```
> wLL <-lm(Weight~DoseLL, data=wuleon)
>
> pN <-glm(Malformation~DoseN, family=binomial(),data=wuleon)
> pO <-glm(Malformation~DoseO, family=binomial(),data=wuleon)
> pLL <-glm(Malformation~DoseLL, family=binomial(),data=wuleon)
>
> wuWeMa <- glht(mmm(covarWe=wN, ordinWe=wO, linlogWe=wLL,
+                    covarMa=pN, ordinMa=pO,  linlogMa=pLL),
+           mlf(covarWe="DoseN=0", ordinWe="DoseO=0", linlogWe="DoseLL=0",
+               covarMa="DoseN=0", ordinMa="DoseO=0", linlogMa="DoseLL=0"))
> Twu<-fortify(summary(wuWeMa))[, c(1,5,6)]
> colnames(Twu)<-c("Model","Test stats", "$p$-value")
> print(xtable(Twu, digits=5,
+ caption="Tukey Trend Test for Joint Modeling of Normal and
+ Binomial Endpoint", label="tab:wuL"), include.rownames=FALSE,
+ caption.placement = "top", sanitize.text.function = function(x){x})
```

Table 5.13: Tukey Trend Test for Joint Modeling of Normal and Binomial Endpoint

Model	Test stats	p-value
covarWe: DoseN	-28.68976	0.00000
ordinWe: DoseO	-30.63006	0.00000
linlogWe: DoseLL	-30.63006	0.00000
covarMa: DoseN	14.64209	0.00000
ordinMa: DoseO	14.24003	0.00000
linlogMa: DoseLL	14.24003	0.00000

All six multiplicity-adjusted p-values (for three regression models, for two endpoints) in Table 5.13 are tiny, i.e., a significant trend reveals for both fetal weight and malformation rate. Ranking the test statistics tells us a stronger effect in fetal weight, both according to the ordinal dose metameters.

5.5   Analysis of female-specific endpoints

Female-specific endpoints, such as the number of corpora lutea (cl) can be analyzed by the nonparametric Dunnett/Williams-type procedure (see Section 2.1.4) because of their count data type, i.e., many tied values occur. As an example the number of corpora lutea from 92 female Wistar rats in an assay with 4 dose groups and a control is used [63]. The two-sided confidence intervals for the relative effect sizes in Figure 5.7 indicate no changes of corpora lutea with respect to control ($H_0 = 0.5$).

```
> data("colu", package="nparcomp")
> colu$Dose<-as.factor(colu$dose)
```

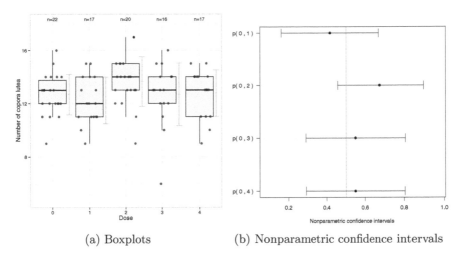

(a) Boxplots   (b) Nonparametric confidence intervals

FIGURE 5.7: Evaluation of corpora lutea.

5.6 Behavioral tests

Behavioral tests are used to identify a possible neurotoxicity. Although a related guideline on developmental neurotoxicity studies with a recommendation of a per-litter analysis exists [285], the particular analysis of such data is not really clear. One reason is that the behavioral data are quite differently structured [142, 141]. Three examples will be discussed therefore.

5.6.1 Behavioral tests on selected pups

A first example is selected where in a neurotoxicity experiment 64 pregnant female rats were randomized to a control and three doses of a herbicide mixture [263]. Upon term, two males and two female pups were randomly selected and used for neurobehavioral testing. As endpoint olfactory discrimination was used (data from Tables 3 and 4 in [316]). The raw data in Table 5.14 contain the factors `Sex`, `Litter`, `Dose`, `Pup` and the endpoint `olfactory`. The hierarchical data structure can be seen from this raw data and from the boxplots in Figure 5.8. Comparing all data (left panel) with sex-specific presentation in the middle (males) and right panel (females), a sex-by-dose interaction can be assumed, i.e., for females a dose-dependent increase can be seen, but probably not for males.

```
> data("ragazz", package="SiTuR")
```

A per-litter analysis can be performed using a mixed effects model with the random factor `litter`. Sex can be either ignored or modeled as a secondary factor (with and without

Table 5.14: Raw Data of a Neurobehavioral Test

Sex	Litter	Dose	Pup	Olfactory
females	1	Control	1	48.24
females	2	Control	1	99.41
females	3	Control	1	31.41
females	4	Control	1	76.81
females	5	Control	1	51.47
females	6	Control	1	42.86
females	7	Control	1	44.63
females	8	Control	1	95.81
females	9	Control	1	18.08
females	10	Control	1	16.13
females	11	Control	1	24.98
females	12	Control	1	16.08
females	13	Control	1	87.55
females	14	Control	1	5.08
females	15	Control	1	41.83
females	16	Control	1	60.92
males	1	Control	1	84.28
males	2	Control	1	16.68
...	...	...	...	...
females	73	High	2	113.28
females	74	High	2	71.26
females	75	High	2	28.31
females	76	High	2	103.45
males	61	High	2	68.22
males	62	High	2	116.34
males	63	High	2	95.79
males	64	High	2	76.88
males	65	High	2	10.76
males	66	High	2	16.14
males	67	High	2	13.05
males	68	High	2	9.71
males	69	High	2	21.97
males	70	High	2	27.26
males	71	High	2	4.13
males	72	High	2	0.65
males	73	High	2	3.61
males	74	High	2	42.30
males	75	High	2	17.16
males	76	High	2	16.64

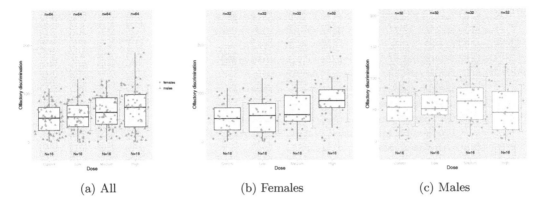

(a) All   (b) Females   (c) Males

FIGURE 5.8: Boxplots for behavioral data.

Table 5.15: Fixed Effect Test on Neurobehavioral Data

	numDF	denDF	F-value	p-value
(Intercept)	1	188.000	562.557	0.000
dose	3	60.000	3.376	0.024
Sex	1	188.000	1.595	0.208
dose:Sex	3	188.000	3.419	0.018

dose-by-sex-interaction) or sex-specific random intercepts within a litter (models mdP1...,mdP5). From the boxplots a dose-dependent variance heterogeneity can be seen. Therefore the assumption of variance homogeneity seems not to be appropriate, and in the related models dP1..., dP5 a dose-specific variance is modeled. Additionally, the naive model of a randomized one-way layout is considered as well (mdPL). By means of Akaike's information criterion the *best* model is selected (in the object myaic): and the winner is the most complicated model dpL5, i.e., with a dose-by-sex interaction, sex-specific intercepts of the litters and variance heterogeneity.

The global F-tests and their p-values in the ANOVA-table (Table 5.15) indicated both a dose effect and a sex-by-dose interaction effect.

```
> library("xtable")
> library("nlme")
> mdPL<-lm(Olfactory~dose + Sex, data=ragazz)
> # litter effect ignored
> mdPL1<-lme(Olfactory~dose, random=~1|litter, data=ragazz)
> # random intercept
> mdPL2<-lme(Olfactory~dose+Sex, random=~1|litter, data=ragazz)
> # sex additive
> mdPL3<-lme(Olfactory~dose, random=~Sex|litter, data=ragazz)
> #  different random intercept within a
> mdPL4<-lme(Olfactory~dose+Sex, random=~Sex|litter, data=ragazz)
> #  different random intercept within
> mdPL5<-lme(Olfactory~dose*Sex, random=~Sex|litter, data=ragazz)
> #  different random intercept within
```

```
> dPL1<-lme(Olfactory~dose, random=~1|litter, weights=
+        varIdent(form=~1|dose), data=ragazz) # random intercept
> dPL2<-lme(Olfactory~dose+Sex, random=~1|litter,
+        weights=varIdent(form=~1|dose), data=ragazz)
> dPL3<-lme(Olfactory~dose, random=~Sex|litter,
+          weights=varIdent(form=~1|dose), data=ragazz)
> #  different random intercepts
> dPL4<-lme(Olfactory~dose+Sex, random=~Sex|litter,
+           weights=varIdent(form=~1|dose), data=ragazz)
> #  different random intercept within
> dPL5<-lme(Olfactory~dose*Sex, random=~Sex|litter,
+           weights=varIdent(form=~1|dose), data=ragazz)
> #  different random intercept within
> myaic<-AIC(mdPL, mdPL1, mdPL2, mdPL3, mdPL4, mdPL5, dPL1,
+            dPL2, dPL3, dPL4, dPL5)
> mod5<-summary(dPL5)
> dPL5X<-xtable(anova(dPL5), digits=3, caption="Fixed Effect Test on
+              Neurobehavioral Data", label="tab:fixNeu")

> fmd<-lme(Olfactory~dose, random=~1|litter, data=fraggaz)
> mmd<-lme(Olfactory~dose, random=~1|litter, data=mraggaz)
> library("multcomp")
> plot(glht(fmd, linfct = mcp(dose = "Williams"),alternative="greater"),
+      main="", xlab="Difference to control")
```

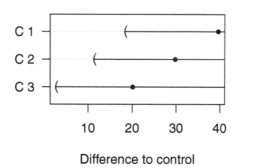

Difference to control

FIGURE 5.9: Williams-type confidence limits for female pups.

Because of this interaction, sex-specific dose-response analyzes by means of a Williams-type procedures are performed; see the confidence plot in Figure 5.9 revealing a clear increasing trend for the females (but not for the males; see the object mmd).

5.6.2   Behavioral tests with time-to-event data

In a second behavioral example time-to-event data are used (see the analysis of censored time-to-event data in Section 3.6.4). The raw data in Table 5.16 show the time prolongation of reflex response such as surface righting after long-term exposure to low electromagnetic fields in the pre- and postnatal development of mice [239]. These censored time-to-event data, i.e., day to first righting, censored where no righting at all occur can be analyzed similarly to the time-to-event tumor data (see Section 3.6.4). Notice, the litter size is not a covariate here, because from each litter 8 pups were selected for the behavioral test.

Table 5.16: Time-to-Reflex Response Raw Data

Group	Litter	Sex	Pup	Day.1	Day.2	Day.3
1	101	m	3	0	1	0
1	101	m	4	0	1	0
1	101	m	5	1	0	0
1	101	m	6	1	0	0
1	101	f	1	1	0	0
1	101	f	2	1	0	0
1	102	m	8	0	1	0
1	102	m	9	0	1	0
1	102	m	10	1	0	0
1	102	m	11	0	0	0
1	102	m	12	1	0	0
...	...	...	...	...	...	
4	419	f	1	1	0	0
4	419	f	2	1	0	0
4	419	f	3	1	0	0
4	419	f	4	1	0	0
4	419	f	5	1	0	0
4	419	f	6	0	1	0

```
> data("frau", package="SiTuR")
```

For these clustered time-to-event data a Dunnett-type test based on a frailty Cox model [158] was used (where group 4 is the control group). Even the large adjusted p-values in the object **ggfr** reveal no effect at all.

```
> cens <- apply(frau[,5:7], 1, function(x) all(x == 0)); frau[cens, 7] <- 1
> day <- apply(frau[,5:7], 1, function(x) which(x == 1))
> library("survival")
> cpfr <- coxph(Surv(day, cens)~ Group + Sex+ frailty(Litter), data=frau)
> library("multcomp")
> cM<-rbindcontr <- rbind("1 - 4" = c(-1, 0, 0, 1),
+                         "2 - 4" = c( 0,-1, 0, 1),
+                         "3 - 4" = c( 0, 0,-1, 1))
>
> ggfr <- summary(glht(cpfr, linfct=mcp(Group=cM)))
```

5.6.3 Morris water maze test using juvenile rats

Learning and memory behavior of juvenile rats can be characterized by selected parameters in the Morris water maze test [269]. As an example we use data for control, low, mid,

Table 5.17: Raw Data of Water Maze Test

group	sex	ano	day	run	latency	time
1	M	1	1	1	9	1
1	M	2	1	1	61	1
1	M	3	1	1	56	1
1	M	4	1	1	61	1
1	M	5	1	1	61	1
1	M	6	1	1	11	1
1	M	7	1	1	59	1
1	M	8	1	1	61	1
1	M	9	1	1	61	1
1	M	10	1	1	23	1
1	M	11	1	1	61	1
3	F	225	1	3	16	12
...	...	...	...	...	...	...
3	F	226	1	3	40	12
3	F	227	1	3	4	12
3	F	228	1	3	3	12
4	F	253	1	3	25	12
4	F	254	1	3	5	12
4	F	255	1	3	61	12
4	F	256	1	3	18	12
4	F	257	1	3	6	12
4	F	258	1	3	40	12
4	F	259	1	3	4	12
4	F	260	1	3	5	12
4	F	261	1	3	8	12
4	F	262	1	3	29	12
4	F	263	1	3	12	12
4	F	264	1	3	15	12

and high dose (denoted as 1,2,3,4) for each 12 males and 12 females of 46-day old rats [113]. The latency times on behavioral tests on 4 consecutive days (triplicate repeated each, denote as run) are used, where the value of 61 sec. represents a constant censoring time point.

```
> data("helena1", package="SiTuR")
```

The raw data in Table 5.17 contains the factors group, sex, day, run where run is hierarchical in day. The factor time represents just 12 runs within days.

Two types of graphical representation are used in Figure 5.10, a boxplot with the sub-units day, run (in the left panel) and a day-by-run-dependency for individual and mean dose-specific values (in the right panel). We see very large between-animal variability, a strong memory effect, i.e., decreasing latencies from day 1 to day 4, a substantial learning effect, i.e., from run 1 to 3 and a related day-by run interaction. On the other hand the dose effect seems to be small and probably not monotonic. This is clearly a one-sided test problem: effects in direction of smaller latencies are of interest only. The latency data represent a time-to-event endpoint with fixed point right censoring at 61 seconds. Furthermore, the dependency between the endpoint and the primary factor dose should be analyzed, e.g., by an one-sided Dunnett-type approach [158]. Moreover, the dependency structure

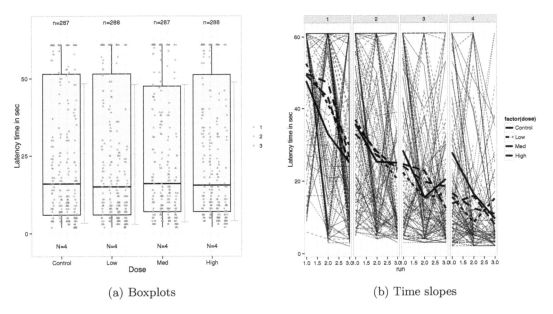

(a) Boxplots   (b) Time slopes

FIGURE 5.10: Water maze data.

of multiple days and repeated runs within each individual animal should be modeled by appropriate random effects. Therefore, a proportional hazard frailty Cox-model can be used, e.g., available in the package coxme. The related p-values reveal no effect at all (see Table 5.18).

Table 5.18: Multiplicity-Adjusted p-Values for
Mixed Effects Cox Model

Comparison	p-value
Low - Control	0.9999
Med - Control	0.9995
High - Control	0.9699

6

Ecotoxicology: Test on significant toxicity

What is specific in ecotoxicological assays? First, dose-response analysis is focusing on potency measures, particularly the no-observed adverse effect level (NOAEL) or the benchmark dose (see Section 7.2). Second, a feasible proof of safety approach is proposed by an authority body, the US EPA [92], denoted as test on significant toxicity (TST). Third, a rather detailed guideline on statistical methods exists [282].

Features:

- Proof of safety using two-sample non-inferiority tests in aquatic assays
- Small-sample size ratio-to-control tests: parametric, nonparametric, proportion

---

6.1 Proof of safety

Some bioassays in regulatory toxicology are carried out to demonstrate the safety of a new chemical, at least up to a certain dose, at least up to a tolerable extent [151, 185]. The non-significance of a common-used point-zero-null-hypothesis test does not represent an appropriate criterion simply because *"absence of evidence is no evidence of absence"* [27]. Here, the proof-of-safety approach [58] can be used where null and alternative hypothesis are interchanged (for a two-sample comparison between control (C) and dose (D) with an increasing toxic endpoint: $H_0 : \mu_D - \mu_C > \xi$ harmful; $H_1 : \mu_D - \mu_C < \xi$ harmless. This specific formulation of the hypotheses fulfills Popper's falsification principle: *we can never demonstrate an effect directly, only by a small probability of its opposite.*

Such a hypothesis test controls the more important false negative error rate directly. Inherently, the *a priori* definition of a tolerable threshold ξ becomes evident. For most bioassays such a threshold is not available. This is even difficult to imagine for assays with multiple endpoints, such as multiple tumor sites in carcinogenicity assays. Recently for aquatic assays, the US EPA defined such tolerable thresholds: for chronic assays $\delta = 75\%$ and for acute assays $\delta = 80\%$ [92]. Specific tests can be formulated, so-called non-inferiority tests [233, 96] (named for an efficacy endpoint in a randomized clinical trial). The advantage of these percentage thresholds is that they can be used for differently scaled endpoints, such as reproduction, growth, or survival. Therefore, ratio-to-control tests –instead of the common difference-to-control tests –are needed (see below). Moreover, a one-sided ratio-to-control test was proposed [92, 94] because the direction of a potential toxic effect is known *a priori*, such as a decreasing number of offsprings. These *inhibition assays* use a vital sign endpoint, e.g., number of offsprings per live female in the *Ceriodaphnia dubia* assay [249].

These inhibition assays are particularly suitable for ratio-to-control tests on non-inferiority, since their continuous, count, or proportion endpoints decrease from large values in the control (sometimes 100%) to small values in the concentration groups as a sign of toxicity, e.g., reduction of the number of offspring. Notice, a second type of endpoints are outcomes of a specific pathological process, e.g., number of micronuclei in the MN assay [176]. The use of ratios in this case can be unstable, because in the control zero or near-to-zero values occur [204]. Still, one-sided tests can be used. A third type of endpoints is outcome of a general physiological process, e.g., serum bilirubin content [19]. A ratio-to-control could be used, but because either increasing or decreasing toxic effects are possible, instead of a one-sided test, two-sided tests, so-called tests on equivalence [185] are appropriate. For assays without *a priori* defined thresholds, confidence intervals can be estimated and interpreted *posthoc*, i.e., up to which amount *harmlessness* can be accepted (see the example below). Therefore, both δ-shifted tests and related confidence intervals are described in the next subsections.

6.2   Two-sample ratio-to-control tests

As a motivation example an aquatic assay on *Ceriodaphnia dubia* [33] treated with nitrofen is used here. In the assay, 50 animals were randomized into batches of 10 and each batch was treated with a selected concentration of nitrofen conc). The number of total life offspring (total) was used as an endpoint, see the raw data in Table 6.1.

```
> data("nitrofen", package="boot")
> nitrof <-nitrofen[, c(1, 5)]
```

Table 6.1: Raw Data of Nitrofen Aquatic Assay

conc	total
0	27
0	32
0	34
0	33
0	36
0	34
...	...
310	5
310	6
310	4
310	6
310	5

In the boxplots in Figure 6.1 we can see the count data. But to the wide range of values between zero and 36 the assumption of normal distribution may be appropriate. Therefore, first a parametric test and parametric confidence intervals are demonstrated.

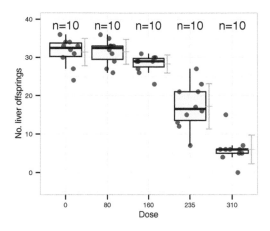

FIGURE 6.1: Boxplots of *Daphnia* data

6.2.1 Two-sample ratio-to-control tests for non-inferiority for normal distributed endpoints, allowing heteroscedasticity

Assuming normal distributed, homoscedastic errors a ratio-to-control test for non-inferiority is available: $t_{i0}(\eta) = \frac{\bar{X}_i - \eta \bar{X}_0}{\sigma \sqrt{\frac{1}{n_i} + \frac{\eta^2}{n_0}}}$, first published by Sasabuchi [337]. This test is central univariate $t_{df,1-\alpha}$ distributed (with the common df). A Welch-type modification for heterogeneous variances was proposed [367, 147]: $t_{i0}^{\text{Welch-type}}(\eta) = \frac{\bar{X}_i - \eta \bar{X}_0}{\sqrt{s_i^2/n_j + \frac{s_0^2 \eta^2}{n_0}}}$ using the Welch $df^{\text{Welch-type}}$. Since a decision-tree approach using a pre-test on variance homogeneity is not powerful, the Welch-type modification can be suggested as default test because of almost similar power compared to the Sasabuchi-test [187]. Even for balanced designs, the Sasabuchi-test behaves rather liberal when in the concentration group a higher variance occurs. This is much stronger, when small sample size exists in this concentration group. The effect even increases with decreasing threshold η [187]. On the other hand, the Sasabuchi-test is rather conservative when small variances occur in the concentration group, particularly when the sample size is small. Consequently, a serious power loss occurs under the latter condition, whereas under the former condition the power increase is invalid. This Welch-type test is numerically available by the function t.test.ratio in the package mratios [121] as well in the software SAS (PROC TTEST). Related confidence intervals [116] were described (formula not shown), and are available in the package pairwiseCI for both homogeneous or heterogeneous variances (suggested as default). The use of two-sample ratio-to-control tests for non-inferiority provides the following advantages: i) use of scale-independent tolerable margins η, which allows their unique *a priori* definition, comparability of different endpoint types and easy interpretation, ii) interpretation of inhibition only, i.e., which concentration still reveals less than a tolerable decrease, iii) higher power in comparison to related difference-to-control tests. The relative efficacy between the test on ratio with respect to the test of difference can be approximated by $n_{ratio}/n_{diff} \approx (1+\eta^2)/2$ [96], i.e., for the 80(75)%threshold the required sample size is $n_{diff} \approx 1.22(1.28)n_{ratio}$ to achieve the same power. Both approaches are explained by means of the above example.

First, separate two-sample datasets containing the control and a concentration group are generated (n080 to n0310):

```
> library("mratios")
> n080 <-subset(nitrofen, Conc=="0"|Conc=="80")
> n0160 <-subset(nitrofen, Conc=="0"|Conc=="160")
> n0235 <-subset(nitrofen, Conc=="0"|Conc=="235")
> n0310 <-subset(nitrofen, Conc=="0"|Conc=="310")
```

Second, four *p*-values for non-inferiority of the total counts in a concentration group relative to the control are estimated (assuming heterogeneous variances and the threshold of 0.75):

```
> p080 <-round(t.test.ratio(total~Conc, data=n080, base=1,
+               var.equal=FALSE, alternative="greater", rho=0.75)$p.value,5)
> p0160 <-round(t.test.ratio(total~Conc, data=n0160, base=1,
+               var.equal=FALSE, alternative="greater", rho=0.75)$p.value,5)
> p0235 <-round(t.test.ratio(total~Conc, data=n0235, base=1,
+               var.equal=FALSE,  alternative="greater", rho=0.75)$p.value,5)
> p0310 <-round(t.test.ratio(total~Conc, data=n0310, base=1,
+               var.equal=FALSE, alternative="greater", rho=0.75)$p.value,7)
```

The four *p*-values are: $p_{80/0} = 10^{-5}$, $p_{160/0} = 2.8 \times 10^{-4}$, $p_{235/0} = 0.99559$, $p_{310/0} = 1$, i.e., both low concentrations 80 and 160 are safe, but 235 and 310 are not *safe*.

```
> library("pairwiseCI")
> fiellertype <-pairwiseCI(total~Conc, data=nitrofen, alternative="greater",
+               method = "Param.ratio", var.equal=FALSE, control ="0")
> plot(fiellertype, H0line=0.75, H0lty=3, H0lwd=1, main="")
```

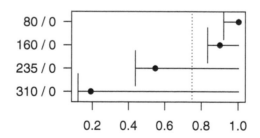

FIGURE 6.2: Fieller-type confidence limits of *Daphnia* example

As an alternative the related one-sided lower confidence limits for ratio-to-control comparisons assuming variance heterogeneity are shown in Figure 6.2.

At a first glance the test and confidence interval decision are the same. But the distance between the lower limit and the $\delta = 0.75$-line gives for 80 and 160 dose a measure of extended safety, in a percentage scale. On the other hand, if a threshold would not be available, we could even claim safety for the concentration of 235 if we would tolerate a threshold of 0.548, which seems to be challengingly liberal.

6.2.2 Two-sample ratio-to-control tests for proportions

In aquatic assays the endpoint percentage survival occurs. Therefore, a related two-sample test for proportions is needed which should be able to: i) model the relative risk as effect size to be compatible with ratio-to-control test, ii) provide a one-sided test or confidence limit for non-inferiority, iii) take overdispersion into account, i.e., not the animal is the experimental unit but the water tank, iii) cope with extremely small samples ($n_i = 3$). Up to now no sufficient approach (confidence limits and compatible tests) is available for these three challenges. Here arcsine transformation for ratio-to-control tests are used [340].

As a data example a *daphnia* assay on copper was selected [43] where the survival rate ($SurvRate = N_{surv}/N_{repro}$) at day 17 is analyzed; see Table 6.2.

```
> data("copper", package="morse")
> copper17 <-droplevels(copper[copper$time==17, ])
> copper17$SurvRate <-copper17$Nsurv/20
> copper17$AS <-asin(sqrt(copper17$SurvRate))
> copper17$Conc <-as.factor(copper17$conc)
> n01 <-droplevels(copper17[copper17$conc %in% c(0, 1.25),])
> n02 <-droplevels(copper17[copper17$conc %in% c(0, 2.50),])
> n05 <-droplevels(copper17[copper17$conc %in% c(0, 5.00),])
> n010 <-droplevels(copper17[copper17$conc %in% c(0, 10.00),])
```

The boxplots in Figure 6.3 show a strong effect at the highest concentration only and some degree of variance heterogeneity.

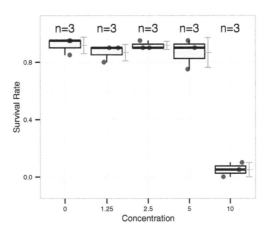

FIGURE 6.3: Boxplots of copper *Daphnia* survival rates

For separated two-sample designs (in the objects n01,n02,n05,n010) one-sided $\rho = 0.75$ non-inferiority Welch-modified Sasabuchi-tests on the arcsine transformed proportions (AS) are used, each at level α:

```
> library("mratios")
> ap01 <-round(t.test.ratio(AS~Conc, data=n01, base=1, var.equal=FALSE,
+                        alternative="greater", rho=0.75)$p.value,3)
```

```
> ap02 <-round(t.test.ratio(AS~Conc, data=n02, base=1, var.equal=FALSE,
+                     alternative="greater", rho=0.75)$p.value,3)
> ap05 <-round(t.test.ratio(AS~Conc, data=n05, base=1, var.equal=FALSE,
+                     alternative="greater", rho=0.75)$p.value,3)
> ap010 <-round(t.test.ratio(AS~Conc, data=n010, base=1, var.equal=FALSE,
+                     alternative="greater", rho=0.75)$p.value,3)
> pvalsAS <-c(ap01,ap02,ap05,ap010)
```

Table 6.2: Raw Data of Copper in *Daphnia* Assay at Day 17

replicate	Nsurv	Nrepro	SurvRate	Conc
A	17	304	0.85	0
B	19	380	0.95	0
C	19	388	0.95	0
A	18	396	0.90	1.25
B	18	485	0.90	1.25
C	16	307	0.80	1.25
A	19	344	0.95	2.5
B	18	285	0.90	2.5
C	18	348	0.90	2.5
A	19	269	0.95	5
B	18	312	0.90	5
C	15	258	0.75	5
A	0	0	0.00	10
B	1	27	0.05	10
C	2	0	0.10	10

The four *p*-values are 0.011, 0.003, 0.044, 0.997, i.e., the concentrations 1.25, 2.5 and 5 are "non-inferior", whereas the concentration 10 is not non-inferior, i.e., inferior (whereas this conclusion can be drawn only indirectly).

6.3   Ratio-to-control tests for several concentrations

Commonly several concentrations (and a zero-dose control) are used in aquatic bioassays. Independent pairwise tests against control, each at level α, are proposed [92]. This approach is not conservative, a serious argument in safety assessment. Two alternative approaches taking all concentrations into account will be demonstrated.

The first is a reversal of the identification of the minimal effect dose under *a priori* importance assumption: if a test on $\mu_{D_k} - \mu_C$ is significant at level α continue with $\mu_{D_{k-1} - \mu_C}$ (again at level α), etc., and stop with the last significant test. The maximal safe dose can be estimated accordingly in a reversed manner [186, 366, 53]: if a test on $\mu_{D_1}/\mu_C > \eta$ significant at level α continue with μ_{D_2}/μ_C (again at level α), etc., until the last significant test. Using the above estimated *p*-values for ratio-to-control tests allowing heterogeneous variances: $p_{80/0} = 10^{-5} < 0.05$, continue with $p_{160/0} = 2.8 \times 10^{-4} < 0.05$, continue with $p_{235/0} = 0.99559$. Because this *p*-value is > 0.05 stop and take the concentration of 160 as maximal safe dose.

The second approach is a simultaneous non-inferiority test based on one-sided Dunnett-type confidence limits, described in Section 2.5.1.

```
> library("mratios")
> maxsd <-round(simtest.ratioVH(total~Conc, data=nitrofen,type = "Dunnett",
+                             Margin.vec=c(0.75,0.75,0.75,0.75), base = 1,
+                             alternative = "greater")$p.value.adj,6)
```

The multiplicity-adjusted p-values for ratio-to-control tests are: $p_{80/0} = 2.5 \times 10^{-5}$, $p_{160/0} = 0.001114$, $p_{235/0} = 0.999969$ and $p_{310/0} = 1$, that is 80 and 160 are safe whereas 235 and 310 are not.

The differences between theses three parametric non-inferiority approaches are delicate. The first (pairwise tests) does not control a familywise error rate, the second (step-up) and third (simultaneous) do. The p-values of the second approach seems to be unadjusted, but they are conditional within a stepup procedure, those of the third are classically adjusted. For this particular example the test decisions from the three approaches are the same.

7

Modeling of dose–response relationships

The majority of approaches in this book are tests on dose-response relationships, such as the Williams trend test. Alternatively, parametric non-linear models for a dose-response relationship can be used. The difference between a qualitative factor dose (assumed in testing) and the quantitative covariate (assumed in modeling) are: i) the relationship between the administered dose and the concentration at the target tissue is commonly unknown, and therefore the less stringent dose level, e.g., zero-dose control and low, medium, high dose may be appropriate, ii) the choice of a particular dose-response model may be more problematic compared with just the assumption of monotonicity when using trend tests, iii) the impact of a particular model function on increased power (in the case of an appropriate model choice) or reduced robustness (otherwise) can be serious, iv) the model fit for designs with only few doses (such as the common 2 to 3 doses) may be problematic. In this chapter three applications will be discussed: i) estimation of ED_{50} (also denoted as $EC_{50}, LD_{50}, IC_{50}$), ii) the estimation of the relative potency between two or more parallel dose-response curves, and iii) the estimation of the benchmark dose (BMD) together with its lower confidence limits. The choice and fit of parametric non-linear models for both normally distributed variables, such as weight, and proportions, such as tumor rates, are shown.

Features:

- Fitting non-linear models for continuous and proportion data

- Estimating the effective dose (ED_{50}) and its confidence interval

- Estimating the benchmark dose (BMD) and its lower confidence limit

---

7.1 Models to estimate the ED_{xx}

Log-logistic models are widely used in toxicology, where the three-parametric (3PL) (by knowledge-based fixing either the upper asymptote to 100% or the lower asymptote to 0%), the four-parametric (4PL) (assuming symmetry), or the five-parametric model (5PL)(allowing asymmetry) are common:

$$\xi(Dose) = c + \frac{d - c}{(1 + \exp(b(\log(Dose) - \log(e))))^f}$$

where the parameter c, d, e, f are the lower asymptote, the upper asymptote, the ED_{50}, and the asymmetry parameter and $\xi(Dose)$ is the response variable in this 5PL model.

```
> data("th", package="SiTuR")
> C2 <-th[th$center=="C2",]
```

Table 7.1: Inhibition Bioassay Raw Data

dose	response	experiment	center
300	0.5	1	C2
100	0.1	1	C2
30	0.2	1	C2
10	0.1	1	C2
3	2.0	1	C2
1	82.4	1	C2
0	128.8	1	C2
0	120.7	1	C2
0	66.4	1	C2
300	-0.3	1	C2
...	...	...	...
300	-3.8	3	C2
100	-3.1	3	C2
30	-3.5	3	C2
10	-4.0	3	C2
3	-1.7	3	C2
1	18.6	3	C2
0	127.4	3	C2
0	105.3	3	C2
0	97.0	3	C2

As an example cell viability data of a multi-center inhibition bioassay of a selected test compound are used running on replicated micro-titer plates (factor **experiment**) (selected data from the ESNATS project [231]). For this specific inhibition assay, the ED_{10} for center 2 (C2) should be estimated for demonstration purposes (see the raw data in Table 7.1). The question arises whether the super-model (5PL) should be used in general or should we better select a simpler but still appropriate model? If a sufficient amount of data is available, i.e., number of dose metameters, number of replicated and informative values (i.e., near to both asymptotes and the point of inflection), the 5PL model can be recommended. In some real bioassays, dose-response data behave not so perfectly and therefore model selection of a sparse model can be helpful to achieve a stable model for a stable ED_{10} estimation.

```
> library("drc", quiet=TRUE)
> m1 <- drm(response~dose, data=C2, fct=LL.5())
> msel <-round(mselect(m1, list( LL.4(),LL.3()), nested = TRUE,
+                   icfct = BIC)[4:6],1)
> plot(m1, bp=0.05)
> m2 <- drm(response~dose, data=C2, fct=LL.3())
> plot(m2, lty=3, add=TRUE, bp=0.05)
```

Using the function **mselect** within the R package **drc** three pre-selected models, namely the asymmetric 5PL, the symmetric 4PL, and the fixed-one-asymptote 3PL model can be estimated and compared by the Bayesian information criterion (BIC) (where smaller BIC means better model). BIC represents a compromise criterion between model fit (minimal residual error) and complexity (number of parameters). Not surprising in this example,

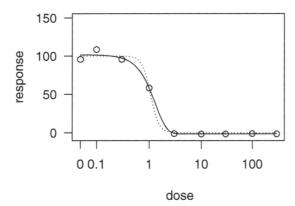

FIGURE 7.1: Inhibition bioassay model fits of 5PL and 3PL model.

the 3PL model shows the smallest of the three BIC values 1772.1, 1776.1, 1779.6: i) the lower asymptote is near-to-zero for this inhibition assay, and ii) no sign of asymmetry exists. Figure 7.1 shows the mean data values and the 5- and 3PL (dotted line) model fit.

Rarely, the objective of dose-response analysis is to identify the most likely dose-response model for interpretation purposes. One should be careful, remembering Box's comment: *" all models are wrong, some are helpful".* More common is the estimation of effective doses (ED). Notice, the ED_{50} is commonly used and also recommended from a statistical perspective because of the smallest confidence interval in the middle of the dose-response relationship. The ED_γ can be estimated by solving the equation $f(ED_\gamma) = \gamma c + (1 - \gamma)d$, where γ is e.g., 50%, c and d are the estimates for the lower and upper asymptotes of the dose-response model. The confidence limits for ED_γ are important because they reflect its uncertainty, and can be estimated by different complex algorithms (not shown here).

```
> ed10 <-ED(m2, c(10),interval = "delta", display=FALSE)
```

In an inhibition assay example, the ED_{10} for center C2 is 0.71 with its 95% confidence interval of $[0, 1.43]$ for the chosen 3PL model. The lower confidence limit of 0 is rather problematic from the perspective of toxicological risk assessment. Already from this example it becomes clear that the confidence limits for other than central ED_{50} estimates are rather wide. This is a contradiction: the narrowest interval exists at ED_{50} while for risk assessment ED_{10} or even $ED_{0.10}$ are relevant with substantially wider limits. When comparing the dose-response curves between centers (C1 - C4) at least two further problems arise. First, to rescale the curves to common lower and upper limits before fitting dose-response models is not a good idea; see details in [389].

```
> m3 <- drm(response~dose,center, data=th, fct=LL.3())
> plot(m3, normal=TRUE)
```

Instead of first rescaling (normalizing) the curves to common lower and upper limits, the model fits of the raw data are performed and then a standardization based on the model fits [324], e.g., using the option **normal=TRUE** (see Figure 7.2).

The second problem is the estimation of relative potency ρ between selected centers. This is demonstrated for centers 2 and 3, because their curves seems to be parallel (a necessary assumption, which can be tested but is not shown here): $\rho_\gamma = ED_\gamma^{Curve2}/ED_\gamma^{Curve3}$.

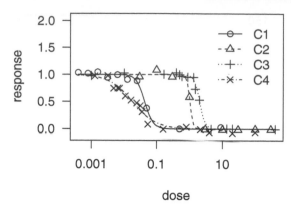

FIGURE 7.2: Center-specific dose–responses of inhibition bioassay.

```
> library("drc")

> th23 <-droplevels(th[th$center==c("C2","C3"),])
> m4 <- drm(response~dose,center, data=th23, fct=LL.3())
> relpo <-EDcomp(object=m4, percVec=c(50,50), interval="delta",
+                display=FALSE)
```

The relative potency between centers 3 and 2 is 0.41, i.e., center 3 reveals that only 41% of the concentration used by center 2 is required to achieve the same inhibition. The confidence limits of $[0.14, 0.68]$ show how large the uncertainty of the estimated relative potency is. Notice, the data are even much more variable, because all the above estimates used the 4 replicated microtiter plates (denote as experiment) and the quadruplicates on the plate as pseudo-observations. Such complex experiments can be better analyzed by introducing a random factor into the non-linear model; see the recent paper [128].

The LD_{50} comes traditionally from proportion data, such as survival rates. A special regression model is needed for such binomial data and commonly a 2PL model is used because for proportions for the lower and upper asymptote the values 0 and 100% can be assumed *a priori*. Here is an example for survival in an earthworm toxicity assay; see the raw data in Table 7.2

```
> data("earthworms", package="drc")
> earthworms$rate <-earthworms$number/earthworms$total
```

Figure 7.3 shows the related boxplots for ordinal dose metameters.

```
> library("drc")
> earthm1 <- drm(number/total~dose, weights = total, data = earthworms,
+               fct = LL.2(), type = "binomial")
> ed50 <-ED(earthm1, c(50),interval = "delta", display=FALSE)

> earthm3 <- drm(number/total~dose, weights = total, data = earthworms,
+               fct = LL.4(), type = "binomial")
> ed503 <-ED(earthm3, c(50),interval = "delta", display=FALSE)
```

The ED50 is 0.15 with a confidence interval of $[0.07, 0.22]$ using the 2PL model. The impact of the *a priori* assumption that the lower asymptote is 0 and the upper asymptote is 100%, is serious. Using a 4 PL model instead, i.e., estimating the parameters for lower and upper asymptote, result in quite different estimates where the ED50 is 0.42 with a confidence

Table 7.2: Earthworm Toxicity Bioassay Raw Data

dose	number	total	rate
0.0	3	5	0.60
0.0	3	5	0.60
0.0	3	4	0.75
0.0	5	8	0.62
0.0	4	8	0.50
...	...	...	...
6.1	0	7	0.00
6.1	0	11	0.00
6.1	0	10	0.00
6.1	1	7	0.14

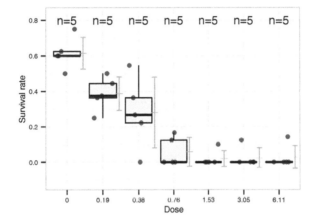

FIGURE 7.3: Earthworm survival data.

interval of $[0.26, 0.58]$. This is not surprizing for these data where no information on the upper asymptote exists; see Figure 7.3.

7.2 Benchmark dose estimation

In risk assessment the benchmark dose (BMD) approach is commonly used. BMD is the dose that corresponds to an *a priori* defined still acceptable effect. Taking the uncertainties into account, its lower confidence limit (BMDL) is used as a point of departure in toxicological risk assessment. This concept is similar to ED_{xx} estimation (and its confidence interval), but the focus is low-dose interpolation for sparse data. Compared with the no-observed-level-dose concept (see Section 7.3 for details) it takes the entire dose-response relationship into account, is less dependent on the experimental design (number of doses, dose metameters, sample sizes, variances), and is based on a biologically motivated acceptable benchmark dose risk (BMR). The BMR is the still acceptable probability of an abnormal response above background (p_0). The two definitions are additional and extra risk [302], whereas additional risk is defined as follows: $p_0 + BMR = f(0, \beta) + BMR = f(BMD, \beta)$ where p_0 is usually specified in advance based on knowledge about the population considered. The definition of extra risk is similar apart from the adjustment of the BMR to pertain to a normal response in the unexposed population: $p_0 + (1 - p_0)BMR = f(0, \beta) + \{1 - f(0, \beta)\}BMR = f(BMD, \beta)$. These definitions stem from binary data, where the BMD concept was developed first. For continuous data these definitions are less straightforward. The risk relative to the variation in the control, the risk relative to the control mean [336], or the risk relative to both the control and the maximum response [273] are used. Among others, BMDL depends seriously on the underlying non-linear model. Using model averaging this problem can be reduced [303]. As a motivating example, part of the developmental toxicity data of 2,3,7,8-TCDD1 is used where the pups affected with cleft palate are considered as proportions to all fetuses (total) (per-fetus analysis) [335] (Table 2A); see Table 7.3.

```
> data("cleft.palate", package="bmd")
> tcdd1 <-cleft.palate[1:5, ]
> tcdd2 <- tcdd1[, 1:3]
```

Table 7.3: Cleft Palate Data Example

dose	affected	total
0	0	325
6	0	95
12	23	118
15	31	65
18	73	103

The function **drm** is used to fit a 3PL model (fixing the upper limit to 1).

```
> library("bmd")
> modBMD1 <- drm(affected/total~dose, weights=total, data=tcdd1,
+                 type="binomial", fct=LL.3u())
> summary(modBMD1)  # background level near 0
> b1 <-round(bmd(modBMD1, 0.1)[,2], 1)
> b2 <-round(bmd(modBMD1, 0.1, ma=TRUE)[,2],1)
```

Using the function **summary(modBMD1)** we see an estimated spontaneous rate of near-to-zero (lower asymptote parameter c) and therefore the BMDL is 10.2 using the function **bmd** in the equal-named package assuming a BMR of 10%. To overcome the direct dependency of a particular model, averaging over a list of models can be used [323]. The option **ma=TRUE** uses an average estimate from 7 models including logistic, log-normal, and Weibull models: a smaller BMDL of 9.9 is obtained.

7.2.0.1   BMD for continuous data

For the more complex problem with continuous data, the number of erythrocytes in hema tology of the 13-week dosed-water study with sodium dichromate dihydrate on female F344 rats is used as a motivating example [3] (see the raw data in Table 7.4):

```
> data("fhema", package="SiTuR")
> fh <-fhema[, c(2,3)]
```

Table 7.4: Erythrocytes Raw Data

Ery	Dose
8.29	0
8.39	0
8.10	0
8.19	0
8.04	0
...	...
9.77	1000
9.41	1000
9.30	1000
9.58	1000
10.08	1000

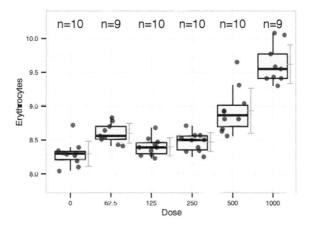

FIGURE 7.4: Boxplots for erythrocytes data using ordinal dose metameters.

The dose-response relationship is not monotonic for low doses (see Figure 7.4), which makes modeling and threshold definition not easy. For the selected 4PL model; see Figure 7.5.

```
> library("drc")
> library("bmd")
> modEry1 <- drm(Ery ~ dose, data = fhema, fct = LL.4())
> plot(modEry1)

> summary(modEry1)
> modEry1$coefficients[2]
> bmdEry <-bmd(modEry1, 0.10, def = "relative", backg=8.4,display =FALSE)
```

Assuming a 10% benchmark risk and a background level of 8.4, a lower limit of the benchmark dose of $BMDL = 190.2$ results.

In a recent publication [197] the BMDL was estimated for both a continuous endpoint (uterine weight) and proportions (dams with malformed pups) using a semiparametric Bayesian joint modeling approach.

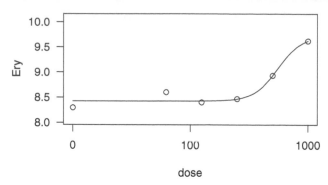

FIGURE 7.5: 4PL-model fit for BMD estimation.

7.3   Is model selection toward LOAEL an alternative?

The concept of estimation of the lowest observed adverse event level (LOAEL) was criticized, because LOAEL depends on the number of doses, their dose levels, and the sample size [236]. Therefore its replacement by the BMD concept was proposed [223]. At least for continuous endpoints we learned from the previous Section that the BMD concept is also not unproblematic. Taking the rather different ways of defining a benchmark dose risk causes different BMD estimates. Therefore, the question arises whether a LOAEL identified by model selection methods instead of testing can reduce the above-mentioned disadvantages. The basic idea of model selection by a generalized order-restricted information criterion is to select the *best* model by an AIC-like criterion, where the number of parameters is refined by a penalty term depending on the number and patterns of inequalities of the particular order-restricted alternatives [232]. This complex approach will be simplified and explained by means of liver weights of dogs in a study on mosapride citrate (available in [411]).

```
> data("fitz", package="SiTuR")
```

Table 7.5: Dog Liver Weight Data

dose	Weight
control	41.9
control	31.2
control	33.7
control	37.3
control	28.3
. . .	. . .
high	54.3
high	38.6
high	34.6
high	39.9

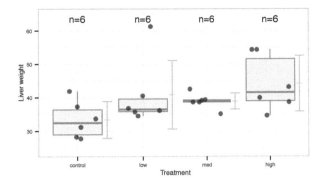

FIGURE 7.6: Boxplots for dogs liver weights.

Figure 7.6 displays the boxplots of liver weight of dogs. The idea is to decompose the global ordered alternative into all elementary alternatives and to estimate specific weights reflecting the relative support of this particular hypothesis in comparison to the whole set of hypotheses using an order-restricted information criterion (ORIC) [232]. In our example with $k = 3 + 1$ doses the global alternative can be decomposed into 7 elementary order-restricted alternatives:

$$H_1^{\xi=1,a} : \mu_0 < \mu_1 = \mu_2 = \mu_3$$
$$H_1^{\xi=1,h} : \mu_0 < \mu_1 < \mu_2 = \mu_3$$
$$H_1^{\xi=1,c} : \mu_0 < \mu_1 = \mu_2 < \mu_3$$
$$H_1^{\xi=1,d} : \mu_0 < \mu_1 < \mu_2 < \mu_3$$
$$H_1^{\xi=2,a} : \mu_0 = \mu_1 < \mu_2 = \mu_3$$
$$H_1^{\xi=2,b} : \mu_0 = \mu_1 < \mu_2 < \mu_3$$
$$H_1^{\xi=3,a} : \mu_0 = \mu_1 = \mu_2 < \mu_3$$

and the global null model

$$H_0 : \mu_0 = \mu_1 = \mu_2 = \mu_3$$

```
> library("goric")
> Cmat_1a <- rbind(
+ c(0, 1, -1, 0), # \mu_1 = \mu_2
+ c(0, 0, 1, -1), # \mu_2 = \mu_3
+ c(-1, 1, 0, 0)  # \mu_0 < \mu_1 <=> -\mu_0 + \mu_1 > 0
+ )
> nec_1a = 2 # The first two restrictions are equality restrictions
> #and the third one is an inequality restriction.
> fm1a <- orlm(Weight~dose-1, data=fitz, constr=Cmat_1a,
+              rhs=rep(0, nrow(Cmat_1a)), nec=nec_1a)
>
> # \[ H_1^{\xi=1,b}:\mu_0 < \mu_1< \mu_2= \mu_3\]
> Cmat_1b <- rbind(
+ c(0, 0, 1, -1), # \mu_2 = \mu_3
```

```
+ c(-1, 1, 0, 0), # \mu_0 < \mu_1 <=> -\mu_0 + \mu_1 > 0
+ c(0, -1, 1, 0)  # \mu_1 < \mu_2 <=> -\mu_1 + \mu_2 > 0
+ )
> nec_1b = 1 # The first restriction is an equality restriction
> #and the last two are inequality restrictions.
> fm1b <- orlm(Weight~dose-1, data=fitz, constr=Cmat_1b,
+              rhs=rep(0, nrow(Cmat_1b)), nec=nec_1b)
>
> # \[ H_1^{\xi=1,c}: \mu_0 < \mu_1= \mu_2< \mu_3\]
> Cmat_1c <- rbind(
+ c(0, 1, -1, 0), # \mu_1 = \mu_2
+ c(-1, 1, 0, 0), # \mu_0 < \mu_1 <=> -\mu_0 + \mu_1 > 0
+ c(0, 0, -1, 1)  # \mu_2 < \mu_3 <=> -\mu_2 + \mu_3 > 0
+ )
> nec_1c = 1
> fm1c <- orlm(Weight~dose-1, data=fitz, constr=Cmat_1c,
+              rhs=rep(0, nrow(Cmat_1c)), nec=nec_1c)
>
> # \[ H_1^{\xi=1,d}: \mu_0 < \mu_1< \mu_2< \mu_3\]
> Cmat_1d <- rbind(
+ c(-1, 1, 0, 0), # \mu_0 < \mu_1 <=> -\mu_0 + \mu_1 > 0
+ c(0, -1, 1, 0), # \mu_1 < \mu_2 <=> -\mu_1 + \mu_2 > 0
+ c(0, 0, -1, 1)  # \mu_2 < \mu_3 <=> -\mu_2 + \mu_3 > 0
+ )
> nec_1d = 0
> fm1d <- orlm(Weight~dose-1, data=fitz, constr=Cmat_1d,
+              rhs=rep(0, nrow(Cmat_1d)), nec=nec_1d)
>
> # \[ H_1^{\xi=2,a}: \mu_0 = \mu_1< \mu_2= \mu_3\]
> Cmat_2a <- rbind(
+ c(1, -1, 0, 0), # \mu_0 = \mu_1
+ c(0, 0, 1, -1), # \mu_2 = \mu_3
+ c(0, -1, 1, 0)  # \mu_1 < \mu_2 <=> -\mu_1 + \mu_2 > 0
+ )
> nec_2a = 2 # The first two restrictions are equality restrictions
> #and the third one is an inequality restriction.
> fm2a <- orlm(Weight~dose-1, data=fitz, constr=Cmat_2a,
+              rhs=rep(0, nrow(Cmat_2a)), nec=nec_2a)
>
> # \[ H_1^{\xi=2,b}: \mu_0 = \mu_1< \mu_2< \mu_3\]
> Cmat_2b <- rbind(
+ c(1, -1, 0, 0), # \mu_0 = \mu_1
+ c(0, -1, 1, 0), # \mu_1 < \mu_2 <=> -\mu_1 + \mu_2 > 0
+ c(0, 0, -1, 1)  # \mu_2 < \mu_3 <=> -\mu_2 + \mu_3 > 0
+ )
> nec_2b = 1
> fm2b <- orlm(Weight~dose-1, data=fitz, constr=Cmat_2b,
+              rhs=rep(0, nrow(Cmat_2b)), nec=nec_2b)
>
> # \[ H_1^{\xi=3,a}: \mu_0 = \mu_1 = \mu_2< \mu_3\]
> Cmat_3a <- rbind(
```

```
+ c(1, -1, 0, 0), # \mu_0 = \mu_1
+ c(0, 1, -1, 0), # \mu_1 = \mu_2
+ c(0, 0, -1, 1) # \mu_2 < \mu_3 <=> -\mu_2 + \mu_3 > 0
+ )
> nec_3a = 2
> fm3a <- orlm(Weight~dose-1, data=fitz, constr=Cmat_3a,
+               rhs=rep(0, nrow(Cmat_3a)), nec=nec_3a)
> # Unconstrained
> Cmat_Unc <- rbind(
+ c(0, 0, 0, 0) # \mu_0, \mu_1, \mu_2, \mu_3)
> nec_Unc = 0
> fmUU <- orlm(Weight~dose-1, data=fitz, constr=Cmat_Unc,
+               rhs=rep(0, nrow(Cmat_Unc)), nec=nec_Unc)
> modsel<-goric(fm1a, fm1b, fm1c, fm1d, fm2a,
+               fm2b, fm3a,fmUU, iter=5000)
```

The weights for these 7+1 models are given in Table 7.6 (whereas `logli` is hereby a parameter for the goodness of model fit, where `penalty` for model complexity under order restriction). The model with the largest weight (`goric_weight`) is `fm1c`, i.e.,

$$H_1^{\xi=1,c} : \mu_0 < \mu_1 = \mu_2 < \mu_3$$

is the most likely dose-response relationship in these dog weight data (compare the dose-response pattern in the boxplots in Figure 7.6). The LOAEL is the low dose because LOAEL is defined as the smallest dose after an inequality constraint. Using alternatively the one sided Dunnett procedure for heterogeneous variances the high dose would be LOAEL-demonstrating the difference between a model selection and hypotheses testing approach.

Table 7.6: ORIC-Based Model Selection for LOAEL

	loglik	penalty	goric_weights
fm1a	-80.319	2.497	0.179
fm1b	-80.300	2.802	0.135
fm1c	-79.513	2.902	0.268
fm1d	-79.513	3.105	0.219
fm2a	-81.946	2.496	0.035
fm2b	-81.152	2.799	0.058
fm3a	-81.275	2.496	0.069
fmUU	-79.383	5.000	0.037

Benchmark dose, test-based LOAEL, and model selection-based LOAEL estimation have advantages and disadvantages. Further work is needed in order to clarify which method is appropriate to identify a critical toxic dose level (or concentration).

8

Further methods

Three further methods are briefly discussed in this chapter: i) toxicokinetics, ii) toxicogenomics, and iii) interlaboratory studies.

8.1 Toxicokinetics

According to the ICH guideline S3A [332] toxicokinetic methods characterize the systemic exposure achieved in animals and its relation to dose and time in repeated toxicity studies.

Features:

- Toxicokinetics: Estimating area-under-the-curve (AUC) for incomplete designs

- Toxicokinetics: Comparing AUCs

- Toxicogenomics: The Benjamini–Hochberg false discovery approach is used for selected probe sets

- Toxicogenomics: Trend tests for high-dimensional data are shown

- Interlaboratory studies: The similarity of the dose-response relationship between laboratories is demonstrated by Dunnett-type treatment-by-lab interaction contrasts

Proportionality between dose and plasma exposure, time and exposure, or dissimilarity between genders or species can be helpful to interpret toxicological findings [308]. Commonly the non-compartmental approach, such as AUC estimation (area under the curve) is used. When using small animals, such as rats or mice, restrictions in blood volume cause the individual animal to contribute data at some but not all time points, i.e., sparse sampling designs are used. Related methods for estimation and testing for these incomplete data are available [205, 404, 405] which are numerically available in the package PK.

As an example the plasma levels of 6 rats of a selected dose group of a repeated toxicity study are used [206]. The comparison of the AUCs between first substance administration and a second after 14 days is of interest.

```
> data("Rep.tox", package="PK")
```

The data consists of an animal identifier (id), the serum concentration value (conc), the measurement time (time), and the duration of administration (day).

Table 8.1: Plasma Level Data

id	conc	time	day
1	0.46	0	14
2	0.20	0	14
1	0.10	0	1
2	0.10	0	1
1	1.49	2	14
...	...	...	...
5	0.54	7	14
6	0.61	7	14
5	0.55	7	1
6	0.27	7	1

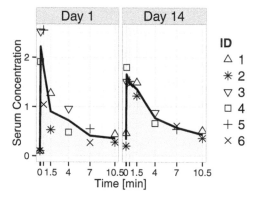

FIGURE 8.1: Day-specific kinetic data.

In Figure 8.1 we see a batch design consisting of 3 non-overlapping sets of 2 respective 3 time points (for details see Section 4.2. in [206]). The AUCs are estimated independent per duration of administration, for the batch design (alternative options are complete or serial design) (their t-distributed confidence intervals are not shown here).

```
> library("PK")
> au1 <- auc(data=subset(Rep.tox, day==1), method="t", design="batch")
> au2 <- auc(data=subset(Rep.tox, day==14), method="t", design="batch")
```

The estimated AUCs are 7.35 for the first day and 8.6 after 14 days of administration. The errors can be estimated as well (and seen via summary(au1)). The question whether the AUC increases with longer administration will be answered by a one-sided test for ratio-to-first day, more precisely the lower confidence limit of Fieller-type interval.

```
> Rep.tox$group <- as.factor(Rep.tox$day)
> ratio114 <- eqv(data=Rep.tox, dependent=TRUE, method="fieller",
+                  conf.level=0.90, design="batch")
```

The function eqv is designed to estimate equivalence limits, but can be used for one-sided test decision by taking the lower limit at a confidence level of 2α. The ratio is $\frac{AUC_{14}}{AUC_1} = 1.17$. Because its lower limit 0.76 is smaller than 1, no significant increase of the serum exposure with longer administration, expressed as their AUCs, can be found. Notice, a special version of Fieller intervals for dependent data are used, because the same animals are sampled at first and 14th day. Instead of ratios, alternatively the differences can be used as effect sizes. Accordingly, comparisons between dose levels, genders, or species can be performed.

8.2 Toxicogenomics

Toxicogenomics is a relatively new field and far less standardized than, e.g., mutagenicity assays. The aim is to select a few biomarkers from *in vivo* studies or to derive prediction models [387] from massively high-dimensional data from *in vitro* studies.

What is specific in toxicogenomics compared to the many recent genomics studies [129, 246], specifically, the use of a completely randomized design, continuous phenotypes, and the focus on dose-response relationships [296, 387] (or even dose-by-time relationships) for high-dimensional endpoints? Related trend tests [311, 242], particularly Williams-type tests [243] and benchmark-dose approaches [44] can be used. As a motivating example the dose-response data of 1000 probe sets (selected out of 11,562) in the dopamine dataset [139] in the package IsoGene [311] is used. For a selected probe-set, namely no. 724, the dose-response relationship is visualized in Figure 8.2. We see an initial near-to-linear slope, followed by a plateau at high doses for a small sample design.

```
> #source("http://bioconductor.org/biocLite.R")
> #biocLite()
> #biocLite("IsoGene")
> library(IsoGene)
> data(dopamine)
> require(Biobase)
> express <- data.frame(exprs(dopamine))
> dose <- pData(dopamine)$dose
> pr724 <-data.frame(respon=as.numeric(express[724,]),Dose=as.factor(dose))
```

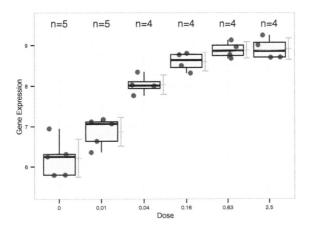

FIGURE 8.2: Dose–response relationship for probe-set 724.

Table 8.2: Raw Data of Serum Creatine Kinase in the 13-Week Study

Response	Dose
6.3	0
5.8	0
7.1	0.01
7.1	0.01
8.0	0.04
...	...
8.8	0.16
9.0	0.63
8.7	0.63
8.7	2.5
8.7	2.5

This univariate problem can be analyzed by the Williams procedure, where the simultaneous confidence intervals for ratio-to-control comparison are presented in Figure 8.3. All five contrasts are under the alternative, where the lower limit for contrast C1 for the comparison of the highest dose against the control $\mu_{2.5}/\mu_0$ is most distant from 1 however less than 2-fold.

```
> library("mratios")
> plot(sci.ratioVH(Response~Dose, data=pr724, type = "Williams",
+     alternative = "greater",conf.level = 0.95, names = TRUE), main="")
```

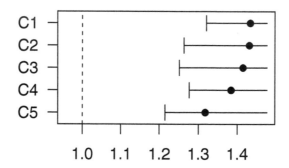

Williams –type contrasts for ratios

FIGURE 8.3: Williams-type confidence intervals for probe-set 724.

Next, all 1000 probe sets are analyzed simultaneously, i.e., first by estimation of the marginal p-value for each individual probe set and then followed by a multiplicity-adjustment method to control the false discovery rate, a common approach in genomics.

```
> library("SiTuR")
> set.seed(1234)
> rawp <- IsoRawp(dose, express, niter=100, progressBar=FALSE)
```

```
> IsoBHPlot1(rawp[[2]],FDR=0.01)
```

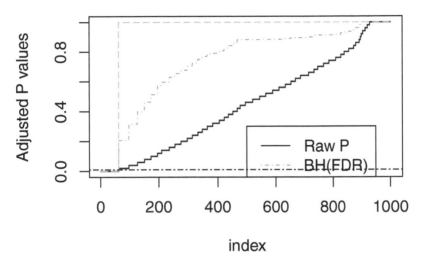

FIGURE 8.4: FDR-adjusted Williams type *p*-values.

Here, the multiplicity adjustment for the 1000 probe-set jointly was performed by the Benjamini–Hochberg approach [30] assuming independent tests, reasonable in this case. The related *p*-value distribution plot is shown in Figure 8.4 for a FDR of 0.01.

```
> set.seed(1234)
> pBHW <-IsoTestBH(rawp[[2]], FDR=0.01, type = "BH", stat ="Williams")
> listTopk <-list(pBHW[1])
```

The top-k-genes are selected where the list containing the significant probe sets in list(207, 227, 235, 257, 284, 311, 332, 336, 352, 358, 381, 389, 439, 443, 446, 466, 478, 492, 501, 565, 607, 608, 624, 649, 653, 664, 677, 685, 698, 723, 725, 748, 832, 837, 886, 897, 925, 943, 944, 946, 953, 988, 989, 4, 40, 110, 128, 135, 199).

8.3 Evaluation of interlaboratory studies

Numerous interlaboratory studies were performed in toxicology with a wide range of intended objectives. Some just compare the global +− outcomes [35], others detailed the similarity of the dose-response curves in different labs [172]. As an example we use the raw data of a rather early stage of a cell transformation assay [166]; see the raw data in Table 8.3. The endpoint number of foci is a count where zero values occur (in lab C even for all control values) and therefore a Freeman–Tukey root transformation is used (see for details Section 2.1.8).

```
> data("interB", package="SiTuR")
```

Table 8.3: Raw Data of Cell Transformation Assays in Three Labs

Lab	Treatment	NoFoci
A	0.00	1.00
A	0.00	1.00
A	0.00	1.00
A	0.00	2.00
A	0.00	0.00
A	0.00	0.00
...	...	...
C	10.00	23.00
C	10.00	20.00
C	10.00	17.00
C	10.00	27.00
C	10.00	20.00

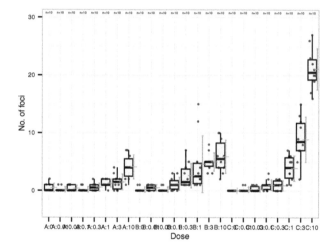

FIGURE 8.5: Boxplots of treatment-by-lab interaction.

The boxplot for the dose-by-lab interaction shows in Figure 8.5 a certain degree of non-similarity of the dose-response pattern (on ordinal dose metameters).

The p-value for the F-test on global interaction in the two-way ANOVA model is rather small (0) and tells us extreme dose-by-lab interaction.

Table 8.4: Multiplicity-Adjusted p-Values for Treatment-by-Lab Interaction

	Comparison	p-value
1	((0.01 - 0):B) - ((0.01 - 0):A)	0.846
2	((0.01 - 0):C) - ((0.01 - 0):A)	0.273
3	((0.01 - 0):C) - ((0.01 - 0):B)	0.997
4	((0.03 - 0):B) - ((0.03 - 0):A)	0.016
5	((0.03 - 0):C) - ((0.03 - 0):A)	0.475
6	((0.03 - 0):C) - ((0.03 - 0):B)	0.000
7	((0.1 - 0):B) - ((0.1 - 0):A)	1.000
8	((0.1 - 0):C) - ((0.1 - 0):A)	0.958
9	((0.1 - 0):C) - ((0.1 - 0):B)	0.921
10	((0.3 - 0):B) - ((0.3 - 0):A)	0.515
11	((0.3 - 0):C) - ((0.3 - 0):A)	0.251
12	((0.3 - 0):C) - ((0.3 - 0):B)	1.000
13	((1 - 0):B) - ((1 - 0):A)	0.000
14	((1 - 0):C) - ((1 - 0):A)	0.000
15	((1 - 0):C) - ((1 - 0):B)	1.000
16	((3 - 0):B) - ((3 - 0):A)	0.524
17	((3 - 0):C) - ((3 - 0):A)	0.947
18	((3 - 0):C) - ((3 - 0):B)	1.000
19	((10 - 0):B) - ((10 - 0):A)	0.003
20	((10 - 0):C) - ((10 - 0):A)	0.000
21	((10 - 0):C) - ((10 - 0):B)	0.000

9

Conclusions

For the three major challenges of statistics in regulatory toxicology: i) proof of hazard with a control of familywise error rate (or comparisonwise only) or proof of safety, ii) uniform, but endpoint-specific Dunnett-type comparisons of the control against doses and iii) p-values or confidence intervals to interpret biological relevant changes, this book tries to give an answer.

The methods presented are not recommendations of a white book, but proposals, so thought-provoking. An attempt was made to present fairly complex statistical methods with few formulas, but reproducible with R code and real data from different assays.

Of course, this book represents only a certain amount of progress and development continues. For example, the qualitative and quantitative criteria in assay validation: *in vitro* against an established *in vivo* assay [344] or the use of standardized effect sizes for different endpoints in repeated toxicity studies [115].

Appendix: R Details

A.1 Selected packages containing specific statistical approaches

The following packages are used in this book:

multcomp [189, 190] Simultaneous inference in general parametric models, primarily for differences between means as effect sizes

mratios [121] Simultaneous inference for ratio-to-control comparisons

drc [324] Analysis of dose-response curve data

pairwiseCI [341] Confidence intervals for two sample comparisons

nparcomp [230] Multiple comparisons and simultaneous confidence intervals for the nonparametric relative contrast effects

MCPAN [342] Multiple comparisons using normal approximation

coin [194] A class of permutation tests

binMto [349] Asymptotic simultaneous confidence intervals for proportions

ETC [148] Claiming equivalence to control

statin [216] Analysis of statistical interactions using contrasts

bmd [322] Benchmark dose analysis for dose-response data

goric [126] Generalized order-restricted information criterion

mcprofile [124] Simultaneous small sample inference for linear combinations of GLM parameters

mmcp [127] Multiple comparisons for multinomial models

PK [206] Non-compartmental pharmacokinetics

nlme [306] Linear and nonlinear mixed effects models

sandwich [415] Robust covariance matrix estimators

survival [373] Survival analysis

coxme [374] Mixed effects Cox models

SimComp [149] Simultaneous comparisons for multiple endpoints

IsoGene [241] Testing for monotonic relationship between gene expression and doses in a microarray experiment

qcc [351] Quality control charts

flexmix [134] A general framework for finite mixture models

mixADA [343] A complex package containing a class of prediction intervals

A.2 Packages containing toxicological data

boot [69] contains data nitrofen

WWGbook [390] contains data ratpup

VGAM [413] contains data lirat

CorrBin [365] contains data dehp

geepack [161] contains data shelltox

aod [237] contains data salmonella

drfit [315] contains data pyrithione, antifoul, IM1xIPC81

morse [91] contains data cadmium1,2, chlordan, copper

nparcomp [230] contains data reaction, impla, liver,colu

mcprofile [124] contains data cta

SiTuR [182] contains several, particularly NPT data

A.3 Packages containing specific graphics and data manipulation

xtable [86] Export tables to LaTeX

toxbox [293] Boxplots for toxicological data

reshape [397] Reshaping data

ggplot2 [398] High definition graphics

plyr [396] Tools for splitting, applying, and combining data

Before processing the R-code, all packages should be installed in advance, e.g. using:

```
> install.packages(c
> ("aod","bmd","binMto","boot","coin","coxme","devtools","drc",
> "EnvStats","ETC","factorplot", "flexmix","gamlss","geepack",
> "ggplot2","goric","gpk","Inlrcde","IsoGene","lme4","MASS",
> "MCPAN","mcprofile","mixADA","morse","mmcp","multcomp","mratios",
> "nlme","nnet","nparcomp", "ordinal","pairwiseCI","pairedCI","PK",
> "plyr","pbkrtest","qcc","reshape2","sandwich", "survival",
> "SimComp","vcd","VGAM","WWGbook","xtable"))
```

References

[1] Lung alveolar cell adenoma in male mice tumor data provided by Dr. Atiar Rahman of Division of Biometrics 6, Office of Biostatistics, CDER, FDA. 2007. Technical report.

[2] National Toxicology Program. 13 Weeks gavage study on female B6C3F1 mice administered with acrylonitrile (107-13-1, C50215B,5021501). Organ weights. Technical report.

[3] National Toxicology Program. 13 Weeks gavage study on female F344 rats administered with sodium dichromate dihydrate (VI) (CASRN: 7789-12-0, Study number: C20114,TDMS number:2011402. Technical report.

[4] National Toxicology Program. 2 Years bioassay of mercuric chloride on female rats. Body weight data. 1993 (study number C60173). Technical report.

[5] National Toxicology Program. 28 Days immunotoxicity bioassay on mice treated with Chloramine (2000). Technical report.

[6] National Toxicology Program. General toxicology. Short term (05161-03) toxicity evaluation of riddelliine (23246-96-0) on F 344/N rat. Technical report.

[7] National Toxicology Program. Micronucleus assay (A63788) of 5-(4-nNitrophenyl)-2,4-pentadien-1-al (NPPD) - 2608482. Technical report.

[8] National Toxicology Program. Reproductive toxicology. Diethylene glycol dimethyl ether. Study number: TER85061 on Swiss CD-1 Mice. Technical report.

[9] National Toxicology Program. Statistical procedures. Expanded overview (2013). Technical report.

[10] National Toxicology Program. Toxicology and carcinogenesis studies of mercuric chloride (CAS No. 7487-94-7) in F344 rats and B6C3F1 mice. No.408. Technical report.

[11] Test No. 479: Genetic toxicology: In vitro sister chromatid exchange assay in mammalian cells. OECD 23 Oct 1986. Technical report.

[12] U.S. Environmental Protection Agency Office of Water (4303T). Short-term methods for estimating the chronic toxicity of effluents and receiving waters to freshwater organisms, Fourth Edition. Section 13: Test method daphnid. Survival and reproduction method. Table 4. Technical report.

[13] National Toxicology Program. Bioassay of piperonyl butoxide for possible carcinogenicity (CAS No. 51-06-6 / NCI-CG-TR-120). Technical report, 1979.

[14] Guidance for industry: Statistical aspects of the design, analysis, and interpretation of chronic rodent carcinogenicity studies of pharmaceuticals. Technical report, US Food and Drug Administration. Center for Drug Evaluation and Research, 2001.

[15] National Toxicology Program. Toxicology and carcinogenesis studies of 3,3',4,4'-tetrachloroazobenzene. TR-558. (CAS No. 14047-09-7) in Sprague-Dawley rats and B6C3F1 mice (Gavage studies). Technical report, 2010.

[16] National Toxicology Program. Toxicology and carcinogenesis studies of sodium dichromate dihydrate (CAS No. 7789-12-0) in F344/N rats and B6C3F1 mice (Drinking water studies). Technical report, 2010.

[17] National Toxicology Program. Carcinogenicity studies on beta-picoline in F344 rats and B6C3F1 mice. TR-580. Technical report, 2014.

[18] Donner A. and Zou G.Y. Estimating simultaneous confidence intervals for multiple contrasts of proportions by the method of variance estimates recovery. *Statistics in Biopharmaceutical Research, 3:2, 320-335,*, 2011.

[19] O. A. Adaramoye, O. A. Adesanoye, O. M. Adewumi, and O. Akanni. Studies on the toxicological effect of nevirapine, an antiretroviral drug, on the liver, kidney and testis of male Wistar rats. *Human and Experimental Toxicology*, 31(7):676–685, 2012.

[20] I.D. Adler and U. Kliesch. Comparison of single and multiple treatment regimens in the mouse bone-marrow micronucleus assay for hydroquinone and cyclophosphamidecomparison of single and multiple treatment regimens in the mouse bone-marrow micronucleus assay for hydroquinone and cyclophosphamide. *Mutation Reseach*, 234(3-4):115–123, JUN-AUG 1990.

[21] S. Aebtarm and N. Bouguila. An empirical evaluation of attribute control charts for monitoring defects. *Expert Systems with Applications*, 38(6):7869–7880, 2011.

[22] A. Agresti and B. Caffo. Simple and effective confidence intervals for proportions and differences of proportions result from adding two successes and two failures. *American Statistician*, 54(4):280–288, 2000.

[23] A. Agresti and B. A. Coull. Order-restricted tests for stratified comparisons of binomial proportions. *Biometrics*, 52(3):1103–1111, September 1996.

[24] A. Agresti and B. Klingenberg. Multivariate tests comparing binomial probabilities, with application to safety studies for drugs. *Journal of the Royal Statistical Society Series C-Applied Statistics*, 54:691–706, 2005.

[25] B.C. Allen, R. J. Kavlock, C. A. Kimmel, and E. M. Faustman. Dose-response assessment for developmental toxicity .3. statistical-models. *Fundamental and Applied Toxicology*, 23(4):496–509, November 1994.

[26] D. G. Altman. Why we need confidence intervals. *World Journal of Surgery*, 29(5):554–556, 2005.

[27] D.G. Altman and J.M. Bland. Statistics notes – absence of evidence is not evidence of absence. *British Medical Journal*, 311(7003):485–485, 1995.

[28] D.G. Altman and J.M. Bland. Confidence intervals illuminate absence of evidence. *British Medical Journal*, 328(7446):1016–1017, April 2004.

[29] D.G. Altman and J.M. Bland. Practice statistics notes parametric v non-parametric methods for data analysis. *British Medical Journal*, 338:a3167, April 2009.

[30] H. Andersen, S. Larsen, H. Spliid, and N. D. Christensen. Multivariate statistical analysis of organ weights in toxicity studies. *Toxicology*, 136(2-3):67–77, 1999.

[31] P. Armitage. Tests for linear trends in proportions and frequencies. *Biometrics*, 11(3):375–386, 1955.

[32] D.A. Armstrong. factorplot: Improving presentation of simple contrasts in generalized linear models. *R Journal*, 5(2):4–15, 2013.

[33] A.J. Bailer and J.T. Oris. *Assessing Toxicity of Pollutants in Aquatic Systems*. John Wiley, 1994.

[34] A.J. Bailer and C. J. Portier. Effects of treatment-induced mortality and tumor-induced mortality on tests for carcinogenicity in small samples. *Biometrics*, 44(2):417–431, 1988.

[35] J.S. Ball, D.B. Stedman, J. M. Hillegass, C.X. Zhang, J. Panzica-Kelly, and A. et al. Coburn. Fishing for teratogens: A consortium effort for a harmonized zebrafish developmental toxicology assay. *Toxicological Sciences*, 139(1):210–219, May 2014.

[36] D.J. Bartholomew. A test of homogeneity for ordered alternatives. *Biometrika*, 46(1-2):36–48, 1959.

[37] P. Bauer, J. Rohmel, W. Maurer, and L. Hothorn. Testing strategies in multi-dose experiments including active control. *Statistics in Medicine*, 17(18):2133–2146, 1998.

[38] F.A. Beland, P.W. Mellick, G.R. Olson, M.C.B. Mendoza, M.M. Marques, and D.R. Doerge. Carcinogenicity of acrylamide in b6c3f(1) mice and f344/n rats from a 2-year drinking water exposure. *Food and Chemical Toxicology*, 51:149–159, 2013.

[39] Y. Benjamini and Y. Hochberg. Controlling the false discovery rate: a practical and powerful approach to multiple testing. *Journal of the Royal Statistical Society Series B-Statistical Methodology*, 57(1):289–300, 1995.

[40] R. L. Berger and J. C. Hsu. Bioequivalence trials, intersection-union tests and equivalence confidence sets. *Statistical Science*, 11(4):283–302, 1996.

[41] G. S. Bieler and R. L. Williams. Ratio estimates, the delta method, and quantal response tests for increased carcinogenicity. *Biometrics*, 49(3):793–801, 1993.

[42] E. Biesheuvel. EMA Workshop on Multiplicity Issues in Clinical Trials 16 November 2012, EMA, London, UK. 2012.

[43] E. Billoir, M.L. Delignette-Muller, A.R. R. Pery, and S. Charles. A Bayesian approach to analyzing ecotoxicological data. *Environmental Science & Technology*, 42(23):8978–8984, 2008.

[44] M. B. Black, B. B. Parks, L. Pluta, T. M. Chu, B. C. Allen, R. D. Wolfinger, and R. S. Thomas. Comparison of microarrays and RNA-Seq for gene expression analyses of dose-response experiments. *Toxicological Sciences*, 137(2):385–403, 2014.

[45] J. M. Bland. The tyranny of power: Is there a better way to calculate sample size? *British Medical Journal*, 339:b3985, 2009.

[46] J. M. Bland and D. G. Altman. Practice statistics notes analysis of continuous data from small samples. *British Medical Journal*, 338:a3166, 2009.

[47] E. Bofinger and M. Bofinger. Equivalence with respect to a control: Stepwise tests. *Journal of the Royal Statistical Society B*, 57(4):721–733, 1995.

[48] J. A. Bogoni, N. Armiliato, C. T. Araldi-Favassa, and V. H. Techio. Genotoxicity in Astyanax bimaculatus (twospot astyanax) exposed to the waters of Engano River (Brazil) as determined by micronucleus tests in erythrocytes. *Archives of Environmental Contamination and Toxicology*, 66(3):441–449, 2014.

[49] J. F. Borzelleca. Paracelsus: Herald of modern toxicology. *Toxicological Sciences*, 53(1):2–4, 2000.

[50] W. Brannath and S. Schmidt. A new class of powerful and informative simultaneous confidence intervals. *Statistics in Medicine*, 33(19):3365–3386, 2014.

[51] F. Bretz. An extension of the Williams trend test to general unbalanced linear models. *Computational Statistics and Data Analysis*, 50(7):1735–1748, 2006.

[52] F. Bretz and L. A. Hothorn. Detecting dose-response using contrasts: asymptotic power and sample size determination for binomial data. *Statistics in Medicine*, 21(22):3325–3335, 2002.

[53] F. Bretz, L. A. Hothorn, and J. C. Hsu. Identifying effective and/or safe doses by stepwise confidence intervals for ratios. *Statistics in Medicine*, 22(6):847–858, 2003.

[54] F. Bretz and L.A. Hothorn. Statistical analysis of monotone or non-monotone dose-response data from in vitro toxicological assays. *ATLA-Alternatives to Laboratory Animals*, 31(Suppl. 1):81–96, 2003.

[55] F. Bretz, T. Hothorn, and P. Westfall. *Multiple Comparisons Using R*. Chapman and Hall/CRC, 0 edition, 7 2010.

[56] F. Bretz and D. Seidel. Sas/iml programs for calculating orthant probabilities for arbitrary dimensions. *Computational Statistics & Data Analysis*, 33(2):217–218, 2000.

[57] J. Bright, M. Aylott, S. Bate, H. Geys, P. Jarvis, J. Saul, and R. Vonk. Recommendations on the statistical analysis of the Comet assay. *Pharmaceutical Statistics*, 10(6, SI):485–493, 2011.

[58] I. D. Bross. Why proof of safety is much more difficult than proof of hazard. *Biometrics*, 41(3):785–793, 1985.

[59] C. C. Brown and T. R. Fears. Exact significance levels for multiple binomial testing with application to carcinogenicity screens. *Biometrics*, 37(4):763–774, 1981.

[60] L. D. Brown, T. T. Cai, A. DasGupta, A. Agresti, B. A. Coull, and G. et al. Casella. Interval estimation for a binomial proportion - comment - rejoinder. *Statistical Science*, 16(2):101–133, 2001.

[61] R. H. Browne. The t-test p value and its relationship to the effect size and $p(x > y)$. *American Statistician*, 64(1):30–33, 2010.

[62] E. Brunner and U. Munzel. The nonparametric Behrens-Fisher problem: Asymptotic theory and a small-sample approximation. *Biometrical Journal*, 42(1):17–25, 2000.

[63] E. Brunner and Munzel U. *Nichtparametrische Datenanalyse. Unverbundene Stichproben. Statistik und ihre Anwendungen*. Springer Heidelberg, 2002.

[64] R. Buesen, R. Landsiedel, U. G. Sauer, W. Wohlleben, S. Groeters, V. Strauss, H. Kamp, and B. van Ravenzwaay. Effects of SiO2, ZrO2, and BaSO4 nanomaterials with or without surface functionalization upon 28-day oral exposure to rats. *Archives of Toxicology*, 88(10):1881–1906, 2014.

[65] H. Buning. Robust and adaptive tests for the 2-sample location problem. *Operational Research*, 16(1):33–39, 1994.

[66] H.U. Burger, U. Beyer, and M. Abt. Issues in the assessment of non-inferiority: Perspectives drawn from case studies. *Pharmaceutical Statistics*, 10(5):433–439, 2011.

[67] F. Cabanne, J. C. Gaudry, and J. C. Streibig. Influence of alkyl oleates on efficacy of phenmedipham applied as an acetone: Water solution on galium aparine. *Weed Research*, 39(1):57–67, 1999.

[68] I. Campbell. Chi-squared and Fisher-Irwin tests of two-by-two tables with small sample recommendations. *Statistics in Medicine*, 26(19):3661–3675, 2007.

[69] A. Canty and B.D. Ripley. *boot: Bootstrap R (S-Plus) Functions*, 2014. R package version 1.3-11.

[70] N. F. Cariello and W. W. Piegorsch. The Ames test: The two-fold rule revisited. *Mutation Research-Genetic Toxicology*, 369(1-2):23–31, 1996.

[71] K. C. Carriere. How good is a normal approximation for rates and proportions of low incidence events? *Communications in Statistics-Simulation and Computation*, 30(2):327–337, 2001.

[72] P. J. Catalano and L. M. Ryan. Bivariate latent variable models for clustered discrete and continuous outcomes. *Journal of the American Statistical Association*, 87(419):651–658, 1992.

[73] P. J. Catalano, D. O. Scharfstein, and L. Ryan. Statistical-model for fetal death, fetal weight, and malformation in developmental toxicity studies. *Teratology*, 47(4):281–290, 1993.

[74] Y. H. Chen and X. H. Zhou. Interval estimates for the ratio and difference of two lognormal means. *Statistics in Medicine*, 25(23):4099–4113, December 2006.

[75] Y. J. Chen, K. C. Lai, H. H. Kuo, L. P. Chow, L. H. Yih, and T. C. Lee. HSP70 colocalizes with PLK1 at the centrosome and disturbs spindle dynamics in cells arrested in mitosis by arsenic trioxide. *Archives of Toxicology*, 88(9):1711–1723, 2014.

[76] Z. Chen, B. Zhang, and P. S. Albert. A joint modeling approach to data with informative cluster size: Robustness to the cluster size model. *Statistics in Medicine*, 30(15):1825–1836, 2011.

[77] R. H. B. Christensen. ordinal—regression models for ordinal data, 2015. R package version 2015.1-21. http://www.cran.r-project.org/package=ordinal/.

[78] C. Clark, C. Schreiner, C. Parker, T. Gray, and G.M. Hoffman. Health assessment of gasoline and fuel oxygenate vapors: Subchronic inhalation toxicity. *Regulatory Toxicology and Pharmacology*, 70(2):S18–S28, 2014.

[79] W. J. Conover and R. L. Iman. Rank transformations as a bridge between parametric and nonparametric statistics. *American Statistician*, 35(3):124–129, 1981.

[80] W. J. Conover and D. S. Salsburg. Locally most powerful tests for detecting treatment effects when only a subset of patients can be expected to respond to treatment. *Biometrics*, 44(1):189–196, 1988.

[81] J. D. Consiglio, G. Shan, and G. E. Wilding. A comparison of exact tests for trend with binary endpoints using Bartholomew's statistic. *International Journal of Biostatistics*, 10(2):221–230, 2014.

[82] D.R. Cox. Regression models and life-tables. *Journal of the Royal Statistical Society. B*, 34(2):187–220, 1972.

[83] G. G. Crans and J. J. Shuster. How conservative is Fisher's exact test? A quantitative evaluation of the two-sample comparative binomial trial. *Statistics in Medicine*, 27(18):3598–3611, 2008.

[84] D. Curran-Everett. Explorations in statistics: The analysis of ratios and normalized data. *Advances in Physiology Education*, 37(3):213–219, 2013.

[85] L.L. Curry and A. Roberts. Subchronic toxicity of rebaudioside A. *Food and Chemical Toxicology 46 (2008) S11*, 46:S11–S20, 2008.

[86] D. B. Dahl. *xtable: Export tables to LaTeX or HTML*, 2014. R package version 1.7-3.

[87] O. Davidov and S. Peddada. Order-restricted inference for multivariate binary data with application to toxicology. *Journal of the American Statistical Association*, 106(496):1394–1404, 2011.

[88] O. Davidov and S. Peddada. Testing for the multivariate stochastic order among ordered experimental groups with application to dose-response studies. *Biometrics*, 69(4):982–990, 2013.

[89] H. D. Delaney and A. Vargha. Comparing several robust tests of stochastic equality with ordinally scaled variables and small to moderate sized samples. *Psychological Methods*, 7(4):485–503, 2002.

[90] M.L. Delignette-Muller, C. Forfait, E. Billoir, and S. Charles. A new perspective of the Dunnett procedure: filling the gap between NOEC/LOEC and EXx concepts. *Environmental Toxicology and Chemistry*, 30(12):2888–2891, 2011.

[91] M.L. Delignette-Muller, P. Ruiz, S. Charles, W. Duchemin, C. Lopes, and V. Veber. *morse: MOdelling tools for Reproduction and Survival Data in Ecotoxicology*, 2014. R package version 1.0.2.

[92] D. L. Denton, J. Diamond, and L. Zheng. Test of significance in toxicity: A statistical application for assessing whether an effluent or site water is truly toxic. *Environmental Toxicology and Chemistry*, 30(5):1117–1126, 2011.

[93] H. Dette and A. Munk. Optimum allocation of treatments for welch's test in equivalence assessment. *Biometrics*, 53(3):1143–1150, 1997.

[94] J. M. Diamond, D. L. Denton, J. W. Roberts, and L. Zheng. Evaluation of the test of significant toxicity for determining the toxicity of effluents and ambient water samples. *Environmental Toxicology and Chemistry*, 32(5):1101–1108, 2013.

[95] G. Dilba, E. Bretz, V. Guiard, and L. A. Hothorn. Simultaneous confidence intervals for ratios with applications to the comparison of several treatments with a control. *Methods Information Medicine*, 43(5):465–469, 2004.

[96] G. Dilba, F. Bretz, L. A. Hothorn, and V. Guiard. Power and sample size computations in simultaneous tests for non-inferiority based on relative margins. *Statistics in Medicine*, 25(7):1131–1147, 2006.

[97] G. Dilba, F. Schaarschmidt, and L.A. Hothorn. Inferences for ratios of normal means. *R News*, 7:20–23, 2007.

[98] R. P. Do, R. W. Stahlhut, D. Ponzi, F. S. vom Saal, and J. A. Taylor. Non-monotonic dose effects of in utero exposure to di(2-ethylhexyl) phthalate (dehp) on testicular and serum testosterone and anogenital distance in male mouse fetuses. *Reproductive Toxicology*, 34(4):614–621, 2012.

[99] J. B. du Prel, G. Hommel, B. Rohrig, and M. Blettner. Confidence interval or p-value? Part 4 of a series on evaluation of scientific publications. *Deutsches Arzteblatt International*, 106(19):335–339, 2009.

[100] J. B. du Prel, B. Rohrig, G. Hommel, and M. Blettner. Choosing statistical tests. *Deutsches Arzteblatt International*, 107(19):343–348, 2010.

[101] O. J. Dunn. Multiple comparisons using rank sums. *Technometrics*, 6(3):241–&, 1964.

[102] C. W. Dunnett. A multiple comparison procedure for comparing several treatments with a control. *Journal of the American Statistical Association*, 50(272):1096–1121, 1955.

[103] D. B. Dunson, Z. Chen, and J. Harry. A bayesian approach for joint modeling of cluster size and subunit-specific outcomes. *Biometrics*, 59(3):521–530, 2003.

[104] G. Ehling, M. Hecht, A. Heusener, J. Huesler, A. O. Gamer, H. van Loveren, T. Maurer, K. Riecke, L. Ullmann, P. Ulrich, R. Vandebriel, and H. W. Vohr. An european interlaboratory validation of alternative endpoints of the murine local lymph node assay - 2nd round. *Toxicology*, 212(1):69–79, 2005.

[105] L. Einaudi, B. Courbiere, V. Tassistro, C. Prevot, I. Sari-Minodier, T. Orsiere, and J. Perrin. In vivo exposure to benzo(a) pyrene induces significant DNA damage in mouse oocytes and cumulus cells. *Human Reproduction*, 29(3):548–554, 2014.

[106] A. Ejchart and N. Sadlej-Sosnowska. Statistical evaluation and comparison of comet assay results. *Mutation Research-Genetic Toxicology and Environmental Mutagenesis*, 534(1-2):85–92, 2003.

[107] M. R. Elliott, M. M. Joffe, and Z. Chen. A potential outcomes approach to developmental toxicity analyses. *Biometrics*, 62(2):352–360, 2006.

[108] S. A. Elmore and S. D. Peddada. Points to consider on the statistical analysis of rodent cancer bioassay data when incorporating historical control data. *Toxicologic Pathology*, 37:672–676, 2009.

[109] M. Elwell, W. Fairweather, X. Fouillet, K. Keenan, K. Lin, G. Long, L. Mixson, D. Morton, T. Peters, C. Rousseaux, and D. Tuomari. The society of toxicologic pathology's recommendations on statistical analysis of rodent carcinogenicity studies. *Toxicologic Pathology*, 30(3):415–418, 2002.

[110] G. Engelhardt. In vivo micronucleus test in mice with 1-phenylethanol. *Archives of Toxicology*, 80(12):868–872, 2006.

[111] W. P. Erickson and L. L. McDonald. Tests for bioequivalence of control media and test media in studies of toxicity. *Environmental Toxicology and Chemistry*, 14(7):1247–1256, 1995.

[112] C. Eskes, S. Hoffmann, D. Facchini, R. Ulmer, A. Wang, M. Flego, M. Vassallo, M. Bufo, E. van Vliet, F. d'Abrosca, and N. Wilt. Validation study on the ocular irritection (r) assay for eye irritation testing. *Toxicology in Vitro*, 28(5):1046–1065, 2014.

[113] C. Faes, M. Aerts, H. Geys, and L. De Schaepdrijver. Modeling spatial learning in rats based on Morris water maze experiments. *Pharmaceutical Statistics*, 9(1):10–20, 2010.

[114] C. Faes, M. Aerts, H. Geys, G. Molenberghs, and L. Declerck. Bayesian testing for trend in a power model for clustered binary data. *Environmental and Ecological Statistics*, 11(3):305–322, 2004.

[115] M. F. W. Festing. Extending the statistical analysis and graphical presentation of toxicity test results using standardized effect sizes. *Toxicologic Pathology*, 42(8):1238–1249, 2014.

[116] E. C. Fieller. Some problems in interval estimation. *Journal of the Royal Statistical Society Series B-Statistical Methodology*, 16(2):175–185, 1954.

[117] P.M. Forster. Explanation of levels of evidence for developmental toxicity. Technical report, US-NTP (http://ntp.niehs.nih.gov/go/10003), 2014.

[118] M. F. Freeman and J. W. Tukey. Transformations related to the angular and the square root. *Annals of Mathematical Statistics*, 21(4):607–611, 1950.

[119] A. O. Gamer, R. Rossbacher, W. Kaufmann, and B. van Ravenzwaay. The inhalation toxicity of di- and triethanolamine upon repeated exposure. *Food and Chemical Toxicology*, 46(6):2173–2183, 2008.

[120] J. J. Gart and J. Nam. Approximate interval estimation of the ratio of binomial parameters - a review and corrections for skewness. *Biometrics*, 44(2):323–338, 1988.

[121] Dilba G.D., M. Hasler, D. Gerhard, and F. Schaarschmidt. *mratios: Inferences for ratios of coefficients in the general linear model*, 2012. R package version 1.3.17.

[122] A. Gelman, J. Hill, and M. Yajima. Why we (usually) don't have to worry about multiple comparisons. *Journal of Research on Educational Effectiveness*, 5(2):189–211, 2012.

[123] A. Genz and F. Bretz. Numerical computation of multivariate t-probabilities with application to power calculation of multiple contrasts. *Journal of Statistical Computation and Simulation*, 63(4):361–378, 1999.

[124] D. Gerhard. Simultaneous small sample inference for linear combinations of generalized linear model parameters. *Communications in Statistics - Simulation and Computation*, 2014.

[125] D. Gerhard, L.A. Hothorn, and R. Vonk. Statistical evaluation of the in vivo comet assay taking biological relevance into account. Technical report, Reports of the Institute of Biostatistics No 10 / 2008 Leibniz University of Hannover Natural Sciences Faculty, 2008.

[126] D. Gerhard and R.M. Kuiper. *goric: Generalized Order-Restricted Information Criterion*, 2014. R package version 0.0-8.

[127] D Gerhard and F. Schaarschmidt. *mmcp: Multiple Comparison Procedures for Multinomial Models*, 2014. R package version 0.0-8.

[128] D. Gerhard and F. Schaarschmidt. *mmcp: Multiple Comparison Procedures for Multinomial Models*, 2014. R package version 0.0-8.

[129] A. K. Goetz, B. P. Singh, M. Battalora, J. M. Breier, J. P. Bailey, A. C. Chukwudebe, and E. R. Janus. Current and future use of genomics data in toxicology: Opportunities and challenges for regulatory applications. *Regulatory Toxicology and Pharmacology*, 61(2):141–153, 2011.

[130] B. I. Graubard and E. L. Korn. Choice of column scores for testing independence in ordered 2 X K contingency-tables. *Biometrics*, 43(2):471–476, 1987.

[131] J. Green and J. R. Wheeler. The use of carrier solvents in regulatory aquatic toxicology testing: Practical, statistical and regulatory considerations. *Aquatic Toxicology*, 144:242–249, 2013.

[132] J. W. Green. Power and control choice in aquatic experiments with solvents. *Ecotoxicology and Environmental Safety*, 102:142–146, April 2014.

[133] J. W. Green, T. A. Springer, A. N. Saulnier, and J. Swintek. Statistical analysis of histopathological endpoints. *Environmental Toxicology and Chemistry*, 33(5):1108–1116, 2014.

[134] B. Grün and F. Leisch. FlexMix: An R package for finite mixture modelling. *R News*, 7(1):8–13, April 2007.

[135] Y. Guan. Variance stabilizing transformations of Poisson, binomial and negative binomial distributions. *Statistics & Probability Letters*, 79(14):1621–1629, 2009.

[136] R. V. Gueorguieva. Comments about joint modeling of cluster size and binary and continuous subunit-specific outcomes. *Biometrics*, 61(3):862–866, 2005.

[137] R. V. Gueorguieva and G. Sanacora. Joint analysis of repeatedly observed continuous and ordinal measures of disease severity. *Statistics in Medicine*, 25(8):1307–1322, 2006.

[138] M. J. Gurka. Selecting the best linear mixed model under reml. *American Statistician*, 60(1):19–26, 2006.

[139] Goehlmann H. and W. Talloen. *Gene Expression Studies Using Affymetrix Microarrays*. Chapman and Hall, 2009.

[140] G. Hahn and W.Q. Meeker. *Statistical Intervals – A Guide for Practitioners*. John Wiley and Sons, Inc., New York, 1991.

[141] M. Hardy and T. Stedeford. Developmental neurotoxicity: When research succeeds through inappropriate statistics. *Neurotoxicology*, 29(3):476–476, 2008.

[142] M. Hardy and T. Stedeford. Use of the pup as the statistical unit in developmental neurotoxicity studies: Overlooked model or poor research design? *Toxicological Sciences*, 103(2):409–410, 2008.

[143] M. Hasler. Multiple comparisons to both a negative and a positive control. *Pharmaceutical Statistics*, 11(1):74–81, 2012.

[144] M. Hasler and L. A. Hothorn. A multivariate Williams-type trend procedure. *Statistics in Biopharmaceutical Research*, 4(1):57–65, 2012.

[145] M. Hasler and L. A. Hothorn. Simultaneous confidence intervals on multivariate non-inferiority. *Statistics in Medicine*, 32(10):1720–1729, 2013.

[146] M. Hasler and L.A. Hothorn. Multiple contrast tests in the presence of heteroscedasticity. *Biometrical Journal*, 51:1, 2008.

[147] M. Hasler, R. Vonk, and L. A. Hothorn. Assessing non-inferiority of a new treatment in a three-arm trial in the presence of heteroscedasticity. *Statistics in Medicine*, 27(4):490–503, 2008.

[148] Mario Hasler. *ETC: Equivalence to control*, 2009. R package version 1.3.

[149] Mario Hasler. *SimComp: Simultaneous Comparisons for Multiple Endpoints*, 2014. R package version 2.2.

[150] D. Hauschke, T. Hothorn, and J. Schafer. The role of control groups in mutagenicity studies: Matching biological and statistical relevance. *ATLA-Alternatives to Laboratory Animals*, 31:65–75, June 2003.

[151] D. Hauschke, M. Kieser, and L. A. Hothorn. Proof of safety in toxicology based on the ratio of two means for normally distributed data. *Biometrical Journal*, 41(3):295–304, 1999.

[152] D. Hauschke, R. Slacik-Erben, S. Hensen, and R. Kaufmann. Biostatistical assessment of mutagenicity studies by including the positive control. *Biometrical Journal*, 47(1):82–87, 2005.

[153] M. Hayashi, K. Dearfield, P. Kasper, D. Lovell, H.J. Martus, and V. Thybaud. Compilation and use of genetic toxicity historical control data. *Mutation Research-Genetic Toxicology and Environmental Mutagenesis*, 723(2):87–90, 2011.

[154] A. F. Hayes and L. Cai. Further evaluating the conditional decision rule for comparing two independent means. *British Journal of Mathematical & Statistical Psychology*, 60:217–244, 2007.

[155] A. J. Hayter. Inferences on the difference between future observations for comparing two treatments. *Journal of Applied Statistics*, 40(4):887–900, 2013.

[156] J. L. He, W. L. Chen, L. F. Jin, and H. Y. Jin. Comparative evaluation of the in vitro micronucleus test and the comet assay for the detection of genotoxic effects of x-ray radiation. *Mutation Research-Genetic Toxicology and Environmental Mutagenesis*, 469(2):223–231, 2000.

[157] E. Herberich and L.A. Hothorn. Statistical evaluation of mortality in long-term carcinogenicity bioassays using a Williams-type procedure. *Regulatory Toxicology and Pharmacology*, 64:26–34, 2012.

[158] E. Herberich and T. Hothorn. Dunnett-type inference in the frailty Cox model with covariates. *Statistics in Medicine*, 31(1):45–55, 2012.

[159] E. Herberich, J. Sikorski, and T. Hothorn. A robust procedure for comparing multiple means under heteroscedasticity in unbalanced designs. *PLOS One*, 5(3):e9788, 2010.

[160] C. Hirotsu, S. Yamamoto, and L.A. Hothorn. Estimating the dose-response pattern by the maximal contrast type test approach. *Statistics in Biopharmaceutical Research*, 3(1):40–53, 2011.

[161] S. Højsgaard, U. Halekoh, and Jun Y. The R package geepack for generalized estimating equations. *Journal of Statistical Software*, 15/2:1–11, 2006.

[162] A. M. Hoberman, D. K. Schreur, T. Leazer, G. P. Daston, P. Carthew, T. Re, L. Loretz, and P. Mann. Lack of effect of butylparaben and methylparaben on the reproductive system in male rats. *Birth Defects Research Part B-Developmental and Reproductive Toxicology*, 83(2):123–133, 2008.

[163] J. L. Hodges and E. L. Lehmann. Estimates of location based on rank-tests. *Annals of Mathematical Statistics*, 34(2):598–&, 1963.

[164] W. P. Hoffman, D. K. Ness, and R. B. L. van Lier. Analysis of rodent growth data in toxicology studies. *Toxicological Sciences*, 66(2):313–319, 2002.

[165] W. P. Hoffman, J. Recknor, and C. Lee. Overall type I error rate and power of multiple Dunnett's tests on rodent body weights in toxicology studies. *Journal of Biopharmaceutical Statistics*, 18(5):883–900, 2008.

[166] S. Hoffmann, L. A. Hothorn, L. Edler, A. Kleensang, M. Suzuki, P. Phrakonkham, and D. Gerhard. Two new approaches to improve the analysis of BALB/c 3T3 cell transformation assay data. *Mutation Research-Genetic Toxicology and Environmental Mutagenesis*, 744(1):36–41, 2012.

[167] S. Holm. A simple sequentially rejective multiple test procedure. *Scandinavian Journal of Statistics*, 6(2):65–70, 1979.

[168] P. M. Hooper and Z. L. Yang. Confidence intervals following Box-Cox transformation. *Canadian Journal of Statistics-revue Canadienne De Statistique*, 25(3):401–416, 1997.

[169] L. Hothorn. Robustness study on Williams procedure and Shirley procedure, with application In toxicology. *Biometrical Journal*, 31(8):891–903, 1989.

[170] L. Hothorn. Biostatistical analysis of the micronucleus mutagenicity assay based on the sssumption of a mixing distribution. *Environmental Health Perspectives*, 102:121–125, 1994.

[171] L. Hothorn and W. Lehmacher. A simple testing procedure control versus k treatments for one-sided ordered-alternatives, with application in toxicology. *Biometrical Journal*, 33(2):179–189, 1991.

[172] L. A. Hothorn. Statistics of interlaboratory in vitro toxicological studies. *ATLA-Alternatives to Laboratory Animals*, 31:43–63, 2003.

[173] L. A. Hothorn. Multiple comparisons and multiple contrasts in randomized dose-response trials-confidence interval oriented approaches. *Journal of Biopharmaceutical Statistics*, 16(5):711–731, 2006.

[174] L. A. Hothorn and F. Bretz. Evaluation of animal carcinogenicity studies: Cochran-Armitage trend test vs. multiple contrast tests. *Biometrical Journal*, 42(5):553–567, 2000.

[175] L. A. Hothorn and F. Bretz. Dose-response and thresholds in mutagenicity studies: A statistical testing approach. *ATLA-Alternatives to Laboratory Animals*, 31:97–103, 2003.

[176] L. A. Hothorn and D. Gerhard. Statistical evaluation of the *in vivo* micronucleus assay. *Archives of Toxicology*, 83(6):625–634, 2009.

[177] L. A. Hothorn and T. Hothorn. Order-restricted scores test for the evaluation of population-based case-control studies when the genetic model is unknown. *Biometrical Journal*, 51(4):659–669, 2009.

[178] L. A. Hothorn, M. Neuhauser, and H. F. Koch. Analysis of randomized dose-finding-studies: Closure test modifications based on multiple contrast tests. *Biometrical Journal*, 39(4):467–479, 1997.

[179] L. A. Hothorn, K. Reisinger, T. Wolf, A. Poth, D. Fieblingere, M. Liebsch, and R. Pirow. Statistical analysis of the hen's egg test for micronucleus induction (het-mn assay). *Mutation Research-Genetic Toxicology and Environmental Mutagenesis*, 757(1):68–78, 2013.

[180] L. A. Hothorn and H.W. Vohr. Statistical evaluation of the Local Lymph Node Assay. *Regulatory Toxicology and Pharmacology*, 56(3):352–356, 2010.

[181] L.A. Hothorn. *Regulatory Toxicology*, chapter tatistical Evaluation Methods in Toxicology, pages 213–223. Springer Heidelberg, 2014.

[182] L.A. Hothorn. *SiTuR: Data files for Statistics in Toxicology using R*, 2014. R package version 1.0.

[183] L.A. Hothorn. The two-step approach - a significant ANOVA F-test before Dunnett's comparisons against a control - is not recommended. *Communications in Statistics*, 2015.

[184] L.A. Hothorn and G.D. Dilba. A ratio-to-control Williams-type test for trend. *Pharmaceutical Statistics*, 11:1111, 2010.

[185] L.A. Hothorn and M. Hasler. Proof of hazard and proof of safety in toxicological studies using simultaneous confidence intervals for differences and ratios to control. *Journal of Biopharmaceutical Statistics*, 18:915–933, 2008.

[186] L.A. Hothorn and D. Hauschke. Identifying the maximum safe dose: a multiple testing approach. *Journal of Biopharmaceutical Statistics 10: 15-30.*, 2000.

[187] L.A. Hothorn and F. Schaarschmidt. One-sided ratio-to-control-tests - simulation results. Technical report, Leibniz University Hannover, Institute of Biostatistics, 2014.

[188] L.A. Hothorn, M. Sill, and F. Schaarschmidt. Evaluation of incidence rates in pre-clinical studies using a Williams-type procedure. *The International Journal of Biostatistics*, 6:15, 2010.

[189] T. Hothorn, F. Bretz, and P. Westfall. Simultaneous inference in general parametric models. *Biometrical Journal*, 50(3):346–363, 2008.

[190] T. Hothorn, F. Bretz, and P. Westfall. *multcomp: Simultaneous Inference for General Linear Hypotheses.*, 2011. R package version 1.2-6, <http://CRAN.R-project.org/package=multcomp>.

[191] T. Hothorn, L. Held, and T. Friede. Biometrical journal and reproducible research. *Biometrical Journal*, 51(4):553–555, 2009.

[192] T. Hothorn, K. Hornik, M. van de Wiel, and A. Zeileis. A lego system for conditional inference. *The American Statistician*, 60(3):257–263, 2006.

[193] T Hothorn, K Hornik, MA van de Wiel, and A Zeileis. *coin: Conditional Inference Procedures in a Permutation Test Framework*, 2007. Package version 0.5-2.

[194] T. Hothorn, K. Hornik, M.A. van de Wiel, and A. Zeileis. Implementing a class of permutation tests: The coin package. *Journal of Statistical Software*, 28(8):1–23, 2008.

[195] J. F. Howell and P. A. Games. Effects of variance heterogeneity on simultaneous multiple comparison procedures with equal sample size. *British Journal of Mathematical & Statistical Psychology*, 27(5):72–81, 1974.

[196] D. L. Hunt, S. N. Rai, and C. S. Li. Summary of dose-response modeling for developmental toxicity studies. *Dose-Response*, 6(4):352–368, 2008.

[197] B. S. Hwang and M. L. Pennell. Semiparametric Bayesian joint modeling of a binary and continuous outcome with applications in toxicological risk assessment. *Statistics in Medicine*, 33(7):1162–1175, 2014.

[198] ICH-E9. Statistical principles for clinical trials. Technical report, CPMP/ICH/363, 1998.

[199] ICH-S2. Guidance on genotoxicity testing and data interpretation for pharmaceuticals intended for human use. Technical report, ICH, 2008.

[200] ICH-S5A. Reproductive toxicology: Detection of toxicity to reproduction for medicinal products including toxicity to male fertility. Technical report, CPMP/ICH/386/95, 1994.

[201] National Cancer Institute. Carcinogenesis technical report series no. 142 1979 bioassay of p-cresidine for possible carcinogenicity nci-cg-tr-142. Technical report, 1979.

[202] R. J. Isfort, G. A. Kerckaert, and R. A. LeBoeuf. Comparison of the standard and reduced ph Syrian hamster embryo (she) cell *in vitro* transformation assays in predicting the carcinogenic potential of chemicals. *Mutation Research- Fundamental and Molecular Mechanisms of Mutagenesis*, 356(1):11–63, 1996.

[203] C.C. Jacob, R. Reimschuessel, and et al. vonTungeln, L.S. Dose-response assessment of nephrotoxicity from a 7-day combined exposure to melamine and cyanuric acid in f344 rats. *Toxicological Sciences*, 119(2):391–397, 2011.

[204] T. Jaki and L. A. Hothorn. Statistical evaluation of toxicological assays: Dunnett or williams test-take both. *Archives of Toxicology*, 87(11):1901–1910, 2013.

[205] T. Jaki and M. J. Wolfsegger. Non-compartmental estimation of pharmacokinetic parameters for flexible sampling designs. *Statistics in Medicine*, 31(11-12):1059–1073, 2012.

[206] Thomas Jaki and Martin Wolfsegger. Estimation of pharmacokinetic parameters with the r package pk. *Pharmaceutical Statistics*, 10(3):284–288, 2011. DOI: 10.1002/pst.449.

[207] P. Jarvis, J. Saul, M. Aylott, S. Bate, H. Geys, and J. Sherington. An assessment of the statistical methods used to analyse toxicology studies. *Pharmaceutical Statistics*, 10(6, SI):477–484, 2011.

[208] P. W. Jones, K. M. Beeh, K. R. Chapman, M. Decramer, D. A. Mahler, and J. A. Wedzicha. Minimal clinically important differences in pharmacological trials. *American Journal of Respiratory and Critical Care Medicine*, 189(3):250–255, 2014.

[209] J. Kanno, L. Onyon, S. Peddada, J. Ashby, E. Jacob, and W. Owens. The OECD program to validate the rat uterotrophic bioassay. phase 2: Dose-response studies. *Environmental Health Perspectives*, 111(12):1530–1549, 2003.

[210] E. Kasuya. Mann-Whitney U test when variances are unequal. *Animal Behaviour*, 61:1247–1249, June 2001.

[211] G. A. Kerckaert, R. Brauninger, R. A. LeBoeuf, and R. J. Isfort. Use of the Syrian hamster embryo cell transformation assay for carcinogenicity prediction of chemicals currently being tested by the national toxicology program in rodent bioassays. *Environmental Health Perspectives*, 104:1075–1084, 1996.

[212] M. Kieser, T. Friede, and M. Gondan. Assessment of statistical significance and clinical relevance. *Statistics in Medicine*, 32(10):1707–1719, 2013.

[213] B. S. Kim, M. H. Cho, and H. J. Kim. Statistical analysis of in vivo rodent micronucleus assay. *Mutation Research-Genetic Toxicology And Environmental Mutagenesis*, 469(2):233–241, 2000.

[214] A. Kitsche and L. A. Hothorn. Testing for qualitative interaction using ratios of treatment differences. *Statistics in Medicine*, 33(9):1477–1489, 2014.

[215] A. Kitsche, L. A. Hothorn, and F. Schaarschmidt. The use of historical controls in estimation simultaneous confidence intervals for comparisons against a concurrent control. *Computational Statistics and Data Analysis*, 56(12):3865–3875, 2012.

[216] A. Kitsche and F. Schaarschmidt. Analysis of statistical interactions in factorial experiments. *Journal of Agronomy and Crop Science*, 2014.

[217] B. Klingenberg. A new and improved confidence interval for the Mantel-Haenszel risk difference. *Statistics in Medicine*, 33(17):2968–2983, 2014.

[218] B. Klingenberg and V. Satopaa. Simultaneous confidence intervals for comparing margins of multivariate binary data. *Computational Statistics & Data Analysis*, 64:87–98, 2013.

[219] K. Kobayashi, K. Pillai, M. Michael, K.M. Cherian, A. Araki, and A. Hirose. Determination of dose dependence in repeated dose toxicity studies when mid-dose alone is insignificant. *Journal of Toxicological Sciences*, 37(2):255–260, 2012.

[220] K. Kobayashi, Y. Sakuratani, T. Abe, S. Nishikawa, J. Yamada, A. Hirose, E. Kamata, and M. Hayashi. Relation between statistics and treatment-related changes obtained from toxicity studies in rats: if detected a significant difference in low or middle dose for quantitative values, this change is considered as incidental change? *Journal of Toxicological Sciences*, 35(1):79–85, February 2010.

[221] H. F. Koch and L. A. Hothorn. Exact unconditional distributions for dichotomous data in many-to-one comparisons. *Journal of Statistical Planning and Inference*, 82(1-2):83–99, 1999.

[222] R. L. Kodell. Should we assess tumorigenicity with the Peto or Poly-k test? *Statistics in Biopharmaceutical Research*, 4(2):118–124, 2012.

[223] R.L. Kodell. Replace the NOAEL and LOAEL with the BMDL01 and BMDL10. *Environmental and Ecological Statistics*, 16(1):3–12, 2009.

[224] J. E. Kolassa. A comparison of size and power calculations for the Wilcoxon statistic for ordered categorical-data. *Statistics in Medicine*, 14(14):1577–1581, 1995.

[225] F. Konietschke. *Simultane Konfidenzintervalle fuer nichtparametrische relative Kontrasteffekte*. PhD thesis, Georg-August-Universitaet Goettingen, 2009.

[226] F. Konietschke, A. C. Batke, L. A. Hothorn, and E. Brunner. Testing and estimation of purely nonparametric effects in repeated measures designs. *Computational Statistics & Data Analysis*, 54(8):1895–1905, 2010.

[227] F. Konietschke, S. Bosiger, E. Brunner, and L. A. Hothorn. Are multiple contrast tests superior to the anova? *The International Journal of Biostatistics*, 9(1), 2013.

[228] F. Konietschke and L.A. Hothorn. Evaluation of toxicological studies using a non-parametric Shirley-type trend test for comparing several dose levels with a control group. *Statistics in Biopharmaceutical Research*, 4:14–27, 2012.

[229] F. Konietschke and L.A. Hothorn. Rank-based multiple test procedures and simultaneous confidence intervals. *Electronic Journal of Statistics*, 6:738–759, 2012.

[230] F. Konietschke, M. Placzek, F. Schaarschmidt, and L.A. Hothorn. nparcomp: An R software package for nonparametric multiple comparisons and simultaneous confidence intervals. *Journal of Statistical Software*, 64(9):1–17, 2015.

[231] A. K. Krug, R. Kolde, J. A. Gaspar, E. Rempel, N. V. Balmer, K. Meganathan, K. Vojnits, M. Baquie, T. Waldmann, R. Ensenat-Waser, S. Jagtap, R. M. Evans, S. Julien, H. Peterson, D. Zagoura, S. Kadereit, D. Gerhard, I. Sotiriadou, M. Heke, K. Natarajan, M. Henry, J. Winkler, R. Marchan, L. Stoppini, S. Bosgra, J. Westerhout, M. Verwei, J. Vilo, A. Kortenkamp, J. R. Hescheler, L. Hothorn, S. Bremer, C. van Thriel, K. H. Krause, J. G. Hengstler, J. Rahnenfuhrer, M. Leist, and A. Sachinidis. Human embryonic stem cell-derived test systems for developmental neurotoxicity: a transcriptomics approach. *Archives of Toxicology*, 87(1):123–143, 2013.

[232] R. M. Kuiper, D. Gerhard, and L. A. Hothorn. Identification of the minimum effective dose for normally distributed endpoints using a model selection approach. *Statistics in Biopharmaceutical Research*, 6(1):55–66, 2014.

[233] L.L. Laster and M.F. Johnson. Non-inferiority trials: the 'at least as good as' criterion. *Statistics in Medicine*, 22(2):187–200, 2003.

[234] R. Lawson. Small sample confidence intervals for the odds ratio. *Communications in Statistics-Simulation and Computation*, 33(4):1095–1113, 2004.

[235] R. A. LeBoeuf, G. A. Kerckaert, M. J. Aardema, D. P. Gibson, R. Brauninger, and R. J. Isfort. The pH 6.7 Syrian hamster embryo cell transformation assay for assessing the carcinogenic potential of chemicals. *Mutation Research-Fundamental and Molecular Mechanisms of Mutagenesis*, 356(1):85–127, 1996.

[236] W. Leisenring and L. Ryan. Statistical properties of the noael. *Regulatory Toxicology and Pharmacology*, 15(2):161–171, April 1992.

[237] Lesnoff, M., Lancelot, and R. *aod: Analysis of Overdispersed Data*, 2012. R package version 1.3.

[238] K. Leuraud and J. Benichou. A comparison of stratified and adjusted trend tests for binomial proportions. *Statistics in Medicine*, 25(3):529–535, 2006.

[239] G. Lewin and T Tilmann. Einfluss niederfrequenter elektromagnetischer felder auf das sich entwickelnde blutbildende system, das immunsystem und das zns in vivo - vorhaben 3608s30006 band 1: Hauptbericht. Technical report, Bundesamt für Strahlenschutz, 2013.

[240] R. W. Lewis, R. Billington, E. Debryune, A. Gamer, B. Lang, and F. Carpanini. Recognition of adverse and nonadverse effects in toxicity studies. *Toxicologic Pathology*, 30(1):66–74, 2002.

[241] D. Lin, S. Pramana, T. Verbeke, and Z. Shkedy. *IsoGene: Order-Restricted Inference for Microarray Experiments*, 2014. R package version 1.0-23.

[242] D. Lin, Z.. Shkedy, and Burzykowski T. Yekutieli, D., H.W. H. Goehlmann, A. De Bondt, T. Perera, T. Geerts, and L. Bijnens. Testing for trends in dose-response microarray experiments: A comparison of several testing procedures, multiplicity and resampling-based inference. *Statistical Applications in Genetics and Molecular Biology*, 6, 2007.

[243] D. Lin, Z. Shkedy, D. Yekutieli, D. Amaratunga, and L. Bijnens, editors. *Modeling Dose-response Microarray Data in Early Drug Development Experiments Using R*. Springer, 2012.

[244] L. J. Lin, D. Bandyopadhyay, S. R. Lipsitz, and D. Sinha. Association models for clustered data with binary and continuous responses. *Biometrics*, 66(1):287–293, 2010.

[245] C.M. Lombardi and S. H. Hurlbert. Misprescription and misuse of one-tailed tests. *Australian Ecology*, 34(4):447–468, 2009.

[246] D. P. Lovell. The use of statistical and quantitative bioinformatic methods in toxicogenomics. *Toxicology*, 240(3):160–161, 2007.

[247] D. P. Lovell and T. Omori. Statistical issues in the use of the comet assay. *Mutagenesis*, 23:1–12, 2008.

[248] S. Lydersen, M. W. Fagerland, and P. Laake. Recommended tests for association in 2 x 2 tables. *Statistics in Medicine*, 28(7):1159–1175, 2009.

[249] R. Manar, P. Vasseur, and H. Bessi. Chronic toxicity of chlordane to Daphnia magna and Ceriodaphnia dubia: A comparative study. *Environmental Toxicology*, 27(2):90–97, 2012.

[250] N. Mantel. Evaluation of survival data and two new rank order statistics arising in its consideration. *Canver Chemotherapy Reports 50: (3) 163-170*, 1966.

[251] N. Mantel, N. R. Bohidar, and J. L. Ciminera. Mantel-Haenszel analyses of litter-matched time-to-response data, with modifications for recovery of interlitter information. *Cancer Research*, 37(11):3863–3868, 1977.

[252] N. Mantel and W. Haenszel. Statistical aspects of the analysis of data from retrospective studies of disease. *Journal of the National Cancer Institute*, 22(4):719–748, 1959.

[253] R. Marcus, E. Peritz, and K.R. Gabriel. Closed testing procedures with special reference to ordered analysis of variance. *Biometrika*, 63(3):655–660, 1976.

[254] R. Marcus and H. Talpaz. Further results on testing homogeneity of normal means against simple tree alternatives. *Communications in Statistics- Theory and Methods*, 21(8):2135–2149, 1992.

[255] B. H. Margolin, N. Kaplan, and E. Zeiger. Statistical analysis of the Ames Salmonella-Microsome test. *Proceedings of the National Academy of Sciences- Biological Sciences*, 78(6):3779–3783, 1981.

[256] C. G. Markgraf, M. Cirino, and J. Meredith. Comparison of methods for analysis of functional observation battery (fob) data. *Journal of Pharmacological and Toxicological Methods*, 62(2):89–94, 2010.

[257] K. Maruo and N. Kawai. Confidence intervals based on some weighting functions for the difference of two binomial proportions. *Statistics in Medicine*, 33(13):2288–2296, 2014.

[258] W. Maurer and and Lehmacher W. Hothorn, L. A. *Biometrie in der chemisch-pharmazeutischen Industrie, Volume 6 (1995)*, chapter Multiple comparisons in drug clinical trials and preclinical assays: a-priori ordered hypotheses, pages 3–18. Fischer Verlag Stuttgart, 1995.

[259] D. V. Mehrotra, I. S. F. Chan, and R. L. Berger. A cautionary note on exact unconditional inference for a difference between two independent binomial proportions. *Biometrics*, 59(2):441–450, 2003.

[260] E.J. Meiman. *Effects on Pinniped Immune Response Upon in vitro Exposure to the Perfluorinated Compounds, PFOS and PFOA*. PhD thesis, University of Connnecticut. Honors Scholar Theses. Paper 362., 2014.

[261] B. Michael, B. Yano, R. S. Sellers, R. Perry, D. Morton, N. Roome, J. K. Johnson, and K. Schafer. Evaluation of organ weights for rodent and non-rodent toxicity studies: A review of regulatory guidelines and a survey of current practices. *Toxicologic Pathology*, 35(5):742–750, 2007.

[262] S.P. Millard. Proof of safety vs proof of hazard. *Biometrics*, 43(3):719–725, 1987.

[263] F. K. Mohammad and S. Omer. Behavioral and neurochemical alterations in rats prenatally exposed to 2,4-dichlorophenoxyacetate (2,4,d) and 2,4,5-trichlorophenoxyacetate (2,4,5-d) mixture. *Teratology*, 37(5):515–515, 1988.

[264] D. F. Molefe, J. J. Chen, P. C. Howard, B. J. Miller, C. P. Sambuco, P. D. Forbes, and R. L. Kodell. Tests for effects on tumor frequency and latency in multiple dosing photococarcinogenicity experiments. *Journal of Statistical Planning and Inference*, 129(1-2):39–58, 2005.

[265] G. Molenberghs and H. Geys. Multivariate clustered data analysis in developmental toxicity studies. *Statistica Neerlandica*, 55(3):319–345, 2001.

[266] H. Moon, H. Ahn, and R. L. Kodell. An age-adjusted bootstrap-based Poly-k test. *Statistics in Medicine*, 24(8):1233–1244, 2005.

[267] H. Moon, H. Ahn, and R. L. Kodell. A computational tool for testing dose-related trend using an age-adjusted bootstrap-based Poly-k test. *Journal of Statistical Software*, 16(7), 2006.

[268] D. F. Moore and A. Tsiatis. Robust estimation of the variance in moment methods for extra-binomial and extra-Poisson variation. *Biometrics*, 47(2):383–401, 1991.

[269] R. Morris. Developments of a water-maze procedure for studying spatial-learning in the rat. *Journal of Neuroscience Methods*, 11(1):47–60, 1984.

[270] D. Morton, P. N. Lee, J. S. Fry, W. R. Fairweather, J. K. Haseman, R. L. Kodell, J. J. Chen, A. J. Roth, and K. Soper. Statistical methods for carcinogenicity studies. *Toxicologic Pathology*, 30(3):403–414, 2002.

[271] U. Munzel and L. A. Hothorn. A unified approach to simultaneous rank test procedures in the unbalanced one-way layout. *Biometrical Journal*, 43(5):553–569, 2001.

[272] F.J. Murray, F.M. Sullivan, A.K. Tiwary, and S. Carey. 90-day subchronic toxicity study of sodium molybdate dihydrate in rats. *Regulatory Toxicology and Pharmacology*, 70(3):579–588, 2014.

[273] J. A. Murrell, C. J. Portier, and R. W. Morris. Characterizing dose-response I: Critical assessment of the benchmark dose concept. *Risk Analysis*, 18(1):13–26, 1998.

[274] J. S. Najita, Y. Li, and P. J. Catalano. A novel application of a bivariate regression model for binary and continuous outcomes to studies of fetal toxicity. *Journal of the Royal Statistical Society Series C-Applied Statistics*, 58:555–573, 2009.

[275] N. Nakanishi, T. Hashimoto, and C. Hamada. Consideration of robustness and power of the Williams multiple comparison test in the evaluation of practical pharmacology. *Journal of Pharmacological Sciences*, 121:68P–68P, 2013.

[276] M. Nazarov and H. Geys. New r routines for facilitating comet assay studies in toxicology m. In *Nonclinical Statistics Conference Brugge*, 2014.

[277] K. Neubert and E. Brunner. A studentized permutation test for the non-parametric Behrens-Fisher problem. *Computational Statistics and Data Analysis*, 51(10):5192–5204, 2007.

[278] M. Neuhauser, H. Buning, and L. Hothorn. Maximum test versus adaptive tests for the two-sample location problem. *Journal of Applied Statistics*, 31(2):215–227, 2004.

[279] M. C. Newman. "What exactly are you inferring?" A closer look at hypothesis testing. *Environmental Toxicology and Chemistry*, 27(5):1013–1019, 2008.

[280] H. Nishiyama, T. Omori, and I. Yoshimura. A composite statistical procedure for evaluating genotoxicity using cell transformation assay data. *Environmetrics*, 14(2):183–192, 2003.

[281] A.M. Nyman, K. Schirmer, and R. Ashauer. Toxicokinetic-toxicodynamic modelling of survival of Gammarus pulex in multiple pulse exposures to propiconazole: model assumptions, calibration data requirements and predictive power. *Ecotoxicology*, 21(7):1828–1840, 2012.

[282] OECD. Current approaches in the statistical analysis of ecotoxicity data: A guidance to application. Technical report, OECD: Organization for Economic Cooperation and Development, Paris, France, pp 62–102, 2006.

[283] OECD407. Repeated dose 28-day oral toxicity study in rodents, updated guideline, adopted 3rd october 2008. Technical report, OECD Paris, 2008.

[284] OECD408. Repeated dose 90-day oral toxicity study in rodents,updated guideline, adopted 21st september 1998. Technical report, OECD Paris, 1998.

[285] OECD426. OECD guideline for the testing of chemicals. developmental neurotoxicity study. Technical report, OECD, 2007.

[286] OECD429. OECD guideline for testing of chemicals: Skin sensitisation: Local lymph node assay. Technical report, OECD/OCDE 429, 2002.

[287] OECD471. OECD guideline for testing of chemicals: Bacterial reverse mutation test. Technical report, OECD/OCDE 471, 1997.

[288] OECD474. OECD guideline for testing of chemicals: In vivo micronucleus test. Technical report, OECD/OCDE 474, 2006.

[289] OECD486. Unscheduled DNA synthesis (uds) test with mammalian liver cells in vivo. Technical report, OECD, 1997.

[290] OECD487. OECD guideline for testing of chemicals: In vitro micronucleus test. Technical report, OECD/OCDE 487, 2006.

[291] J. Ogawa. On the confidence-bounds of the ratio of the means of a bivariate normal-distribution. *Annals of the Institute of Statistical Mathematics*, 35(1):41–48, 1983.

[292] J. G. Orelien, J. Zhai, R. Morris, and R. Cohn. An approach to performing multiple comparisons with a control in GEE models. *Communications in Statistics-Theory and Methods*, 31(1):87–105, 2002.

[293] P. Pallmann. *toxbox: Boxplots for Toxicological Data*, 2015. R package version 1.1.3.

[294] P. Pallmann and L.A. Hothorn. Boxplots for grouped and clustered data in toxicology. *Archives of Toxicology*, DOI 10.1007/s00204-015-1608-4, 2015.

[295] P. Pallmann, M. Pretorious, and C. Ritz. Simultaneous comparisons of treatments at multiple time points: Combined marginal models versus joint modeling. *Statistical Methods in Medical Research*, 2015.

[296] C. Parfett, A. Williams, J. L. Zheng, and G. Zhou. Gene batteries and synexpression groups applied in a multivariate statistical approach to dose-response analysis of toxicogenomic data. *Regulatory Toxicology and Pharmacology*, 67(1):63–74, 2013.

[297] S. Paul and K. K. Saha. The generalized linear model and extensions: A review and some biological and environmental applications. *Environmetrics*, 18(4):421–443, 2007.

[298] S. R. Paul. Analysis of proportions of affected fetuses in teratological experiments. *Biometrics*, 38(2):361–370, 1982.

[299] S. D. Peddada and G. E. Kissling. A survival-adjusted quantal-response test for analysis of tumor incidence rates in animal carcinogenicity studies. *Environmental Health Perspectives*, 114(4):537–541, 2006.

[300] R. Peto, M.C. Pike, and N.E. . Day. Guidelines for simple sensitive significance tests for carcinogenic effects in long-term animal experiments. Technical report, IARC Monographs on the Evaluation of the Carcinogenic Risk of Chemicals to Humans. Supplement 2: Long-term and Short-term Screening Assays for Carcinogens: A Critical Appraisal. Lyon: International Agency for Research on Cancer. 311-346., 1980.

[301] A. Phillips, C. Fletcher, G. Atkinson, E. Channon, A. Douiri, T. Jaki, J. Maca, D. Morgan, J. H. Roger, and P. Terrill. Multiplicity: Discussion points from the Statisticians in the Pharmaceutical Industry multiplicity expert group. *Pharmaceutical Statistics*, 12(5):255–259, 2013.

[302] W. W. Piegorsch. Translational benchmark risk analysis. *Journal of Risk Research*, 13(5):653–667, 2010.

[303] W. W. Piegorsch, L. L. An, A. A. Wickens, R. W. West, E. A. Pena, and W. S. Wu. Information-theoretic model-averaged benchmark dose analysis in environmental risk assessment. *Environmetrics*, 24(3):143–157, 2013.

[304] H. P. Piepho. An algorithm for a letter-based representation of all-pairwise comparisons. *Journal of Computational and Graphical Statistics*, 13(2):456–466, 2004.

[305] H. P. Piepho, A. Buchse, and K. Emrich. A hitchhiker's guide to mixed models for randomized experiments. *Journal of Agronomy and Crop Science*, 189(5):310–322, 2003.

[306] J. Pinheiro, D. Bates, S. DebRoy, and D. Sarkar. *nlme: Linear and Nonlinear Mixed Effects Models*, 2014. R package version 3.1-117.

[307] C. B. Pipper, C. Ritz, and H. Bisgaard. A versatile method for confirmatory evaluation of the effects of a covariate in multiple models. *Journal of the Royal Statistical Society Series C- Applied Statistics*, 61:315–326, 2012.

[308] J. P. H. T. M. Ploemen, H. Kramer, E. I. Krajnc, and I. Martin. The use of toxicokinetic data in preclinical safety assessment: A toxicologic pathologist perspective. *Toxicological Pathology*, 35(6):834–837, 2007.

[309] M. J. Podgor, J. L. Gastwirth, and C. R. Mehta. Efficiency robust tests of independence in contingency tables with ordered classifications. *Statistics in Medicine*, 15(19):2095–2105, 1996.

[310] C. J. Portier and A. J. Bailer. Testing for increased carcinogenicity using a survival-adjusted quantal response test. *Fundamental and Applied Toxicology*, 12(4):731–737, 1989.

[311] S. Pramana, D. Lin, P. Haldermans, Z. Shkedy, T. Verbeke, H. Gohlmann, A. De Bondt, W. Talloen, and L. Bijnens. Isogene: An r package for analyzing dose-response studies in microarray experiments. *R Journal*, 2(1):5–12, 2010.

[312] C. J. Price, C. A. Kimmel, J. D. George, and M. C. MARR. The developmental toxicity of diethylene glycol dimethyl ether in mice. *Fundamental and Applied Toxicology*, 8(1):115–126, 1987.

[313] R. M. Price and D. G. Bonett. An improved confidence interval for a linear function of binomial proportions. *Computational Statistics & Data Analysis*, 45(3):449–456, 2004.

[314] National Toxicology Program. National toxicology program. Toxicology and carcinogenesis studies of methyleugenol in F344/n rats and B6C3F1 mice. Technical report, 2000, Technical Report 491.

[315] J. Ranke. *drfit: Dose-response data evaluation*, 2014. R package version 0.6.3.

[316] M. Razzaghi. A hierarchical model for the skew-normal distribution with application in developmental neurotoxicology. *Communications in Statistics-Theory and Methods*, 43(8):1859–1872, 2014.

[317] J. Reiczigel, D. Zakarias, and L. Rozsa. A bootstrap test of stochastic equality of two populations. *American Statistician*, 59(2):156–161, 2005.

[318] G. Reifferscheid, H. M. Maes, B. Allner, J. Badurova, S. Belkin, K. Bluhm, F. Brauer, J. Bressling, S. Domeneghetti, T. Elad, S. Flueckiger-Isler, H. S. Grummt, R. Guertler, A. Hecht, M. B. Heringa, H. Hollert, S. Huber, M. Kramer, A. Magdeburg, H. T. Ratte, R. Sauerborn-Klobucar, A. Sokolowski, P. Soldan, T. Smital, D. Stalter, P. Venier, C. Ziemann, J. Zipperle, and S. Buchinger. International round-robin study on the Ames fluctuation test. *Environmental and Molecular Mutagenesis*, 53(3):185–197, 2012.

[319] M. Rhodes, S. Laffan, C. Genell, J. Gower, C. Maier, T. Fukushima, G. Nichols, and A. E. Bassiri. Assessing a theoretical risk of dolutegravir-induced developmental immunotoxicity in juvenile rats. *Toxicological Sciences*, 130(1):70–81, 2012.

[320] C. Rigaud, C. M. Couillard, J. Pellerin, B. Legare, and P. V. Hodson. Applicability of the TCDD-TEQ approach to predict sublethal embryo-toxicity in Fundulus heteroclitus. *Aquatic Toxicology*, 149:133–144, 2014.

[321] R. A. Rigby and D. M. Stasinopoulos. Generalized additive models for location, scale and shape. *Journal of the Royal Statistical Society Series C- Applied Statistics*, 54:507–544, 2005.

[322] C. Ritz. Benchmark Dose Analysis in R. Under preparation, 2009.

[323] C. Ritz, D. Gerhard, and L. A. Hothorn. A unified framework for benchmark dose estimation applied to mixed models and model averaging. *Statistics in Biopharmaceutical Research*, 5(1):79–90, 2013.

[324] C. Ritz and J. C. Streibig. Bioassay Analysis using R. *Journal of Statistical Software*, 12, 2005.

[325] C. Ritz and L. Van der Vliet. Handling nonnormality and variance heterogeneity for quantitative sublethal toxicity tests. *Environmental Toxicology and Chemistry*, 28(9):2009–2017, 2009.

[326] M. Royer, P. N. Diouf, and T. Stevanovic. Polyphenol contents and radical scavenging capacities of red maple (acer rubrum l.) extracts. *Food and Chemical Toxicology*, 49(9):2180–2188, 2011.

[327] G. Rucker, G. Schwarzer, J. Carpenter, and I. Olkin. Why add anything to nothing? the arcsine difference as a measure of treatment effect in meta-analysis with zero cells. *Statistics in Medicine*, 28(5):721–738, 2009.

[328] P. E. Rudolph. Robustness of multiple comparison procedures - treatment versus control. *Biometrical Journal*, 30(1):41–45, 1988.

[329] G. D. Ruxton. The unequal variance t-test is an underused alternative to Student's t-test and the Mann-Whitney U test. *Behavioral Ecology*, 17(4):688–690, 2006.

[330] E. Ryu. Simultaneous confidence intervals using ordinal effect measures for ordered categorical outcomes. *Statistics in Medicine*, 28(25):3179–3188, 2009.

[331] E. J. Ryu and A. Agresti. Modeling and inference for an ordinal effect size measure. *Statistics in Medicine*, 27(10):1703–1717, 2008.

[332] ICH S3a. Note for guidance on toxicokinetics: A guidance for assessing systemic exposure in toxicology studies (cpmp/ich/384/95). Technical report, CPMP/ICH, 1995.

[333] K. K. Saha, R. Bilisoly, and D. M. Dziuda. Hybrid-based confidence intervals for the ratio of two treatment means in the over-dispersed Poisson data. *Journal of Applied Statistics*, 41(2):439–453, 2014.

[334] K.K. Saha. Inference concerning a common dispersion of several treatment groups in the analysis of over/underdispersed count data. *Biometrical Journal*, 56(3):441–460, 2014.

[335] S. Sand, A. F. Filipsson, and K. Victorin. Evaluation of the benchmark dose method for dichotomous data: Model dependence and model selection. *Regulatory Toxicology and Pharmacology*, 36(2):184–197, 2002.

[336] S. Sand, D. von Rosen, P. Eriksson, A. Fredriksson, H. Viberg, K. Victorin, and A. F. Filipsson. Dose-response modeling and benchmark calculations from spontaneous behavior data on mice neonatally exposed to 2,2 ',4,4 ',5-pentabromodiphenyl ether. *Toxicological Sciences*, 81(2):491–501, 2004.

[337] S. Sasabuchi. A multivariate one-sided test with composite hypothesis when the covariance matrix is completely unknown. *Memoirs of the Faculty of Science, Series A*, 42:37–46, 1988.

[338] F. Schaarschmidt. Simultaneous confidence intervals for multiple comparisons among expected values of log-normal variables. *Computational Statistics and Data Analysis*, 58:265–275, 2013.

[339] F. Schaarschmidt. *mixADA: Normalization, mixture models and screening cutpoints for anti-drug-antibody reactions (based on contributions by Bettina Gruen and Thomas Jaki and Ludwig Hothorn)*, 2014. R package version 1.2.

[340] F Schaarschmidt. One-sided ratio-to-control tests - simulation results. Technical report, Leibniz University Hannover. Institute of Biostatistics, 2014.

[341] F. Schaarschmidt and D. Gerhard. *pairwiseCI: Confidence intervals for two sample comparisons*, 2013. R package version 0.1-22.

[342] F. Schaarschmidt, D. Gerhard, and M. Sill. *MCPAN: Multiple comparisons using normal approximation*, 2013. R package version 1.1-15.

[343] F. Schaarschmidt, M. Hofmann, T. Jaki, B. Gruen, and L. A. Hothorn. Statistical approaches for the determination of cut points in anti-drug antibody bioassays. *Journal of Immunological Methods*, 418:84–100, 2015.

[344] F. Schaarschmidt and L. A. Hothorn. Statistical methods and software for validation studies on new in vitro toxicity assays. *ATLA-Alternatives to Laboratory Animals*, 42(5):318–325, November 2014.

[345] F. Schaarschmidt and L.A. Hothorn. A note on prediction intervals for comparisons of a future group of historical control data. Technical report, Reports of the Institute of Biostatistics 01/2015. Leibniz University Hannover, 2015.

[346] F. Schaarschmidt, M. Sill, and L. A. Hothorn. Approximate Simultaneous Confidence Intervals for Multiple Contrasts of Binomial Proportions. *Biometrical Journal*, 50(5, SI):782–792, OCT 2008.

[347] F. Schaarschmidt, M. Sill, and L. A. Hothorn. Poly-k-trend tests for survival adjusted analysis of tumor rates formulated as approximate multiple contrast test. *Journal of Biopharmaceutical Statistics*, 18(5):934–948, 2008.

[348] F. Schaarschmidt and L. Vaas. Analysis of trials with complex treatment structure using multiple contrast tests. *Hortscience*, 44(1):188–195, 2009.

[349] Frank Schaarschmidt. *binMto: Asymptotic simultaneous confidence intervals for many-to-one comparisons of proportions*, 2013. R package version 0.0-6.

[350] M. Scholze and A. Kortenkamp. Statistical power considerations show the endocrine disruptor low-dose issue in a new light. *Environmental Health Perspectives*, 115:84–90, 2007.

[351] L. Scrucca. qcc: an R package for quality control charting and statistical process control. *R News*, 4/1:11–17, 2004.

[352] D. Seidel. *Trendtests für geordnete kategoriale Daten bei sehr kleinen Fallzahlen*. PhD thesis, University of Hannover, 1999.

[353] R. S. Sellers, D. Morton, B. Michael, N. Roome, J. K. Johnson, B. L. Yano, R. Perry, and K. Schafer. Society of toxicologic pathology position paper: Organ weight recommendations for toxicology studies. *Toxicologic Pathology*, 35(5):751–755, 2007.

[354] S. Senn. Change from baseline and analysis of covariance revisited. *Statistics in Medicine*, 25(24):4334–4344, 2006.

[355] E. A. C. Shirley and P. Newham. The choice between analysis of variance and analysis of covariance with special reference to the analysis of organ weights in toxicology studies. *Statistics in Medicine*, 3(1):85–91, 1984.

[356] E.A.C. Shirley. A nonparametric equivalent of Williams' test for contrasting increasing dose levels of a treatment. *Biometrics*, 33(2):386–389, 1977.

[357] C. H. Sim, F. F. Gan, and T. C. Chang. Outlier labeling with boxplot procedures. *Journal of the American Statistical Association*, 100(470):642–652, 2005.

[358] R. T. Smythe, D. Krewski, and D. Murdoch. The use of historical control information in modeling dose-response relationships in carcinogenesis. *Statistics & Probability Letters*, 4(2):87–93, 1986.

[359] E. Sonnemann. General solutions to multiple testing problems. *Biometrical Journal*, 50(5, SI):641–656, 2008.

[360] M. Sprengel. *Analyse kategorialer Daten mit speziellem Fokus auf simultane Konfidenzintervalle*. PhD thesis, MASTERARBEIT zur Erlangung des Grades eines M.Sc. der Gartenbauwissenschaften der naturwissenschaftlichen Fakultaet an der Leipniz Universitaet Hannover, 2011.

[361] D. M. Stasinopoulos and R. A. Rigby. Generalized additive models for location scale and shape (gamlss) in r. *Journal of Statistical Software*, 23(7), 2007.

[362] K. E. Stebbins, K. A. Johnson, T. K. Jeffries, J. M. Redmond, K. T. Haut, S. N. Shabrang, and W. T. Stott. Chronic toxicity and oncogenicity studies of ingested 1,3-dichloropropene in rats and mice. *Regulatory Toxicology And Pharmacology*, 32(1):1–13, 2000.

[363] O. Sverdlov and W.Kee. Wong. Novel statistical designs for phase I/II and phase II clinical trials with dose-finding objectives. *Therapeutic Innovation & Regulatory Science*, 48(5):601–612, 2014.

[364] A. Swain, J. Turton, and C. et al. Scudamore. Nephrotoxicity of hexachloro-1:3-butadiene in the male Hanover Wistar rat; correlation of minimal histopathological changes with biomarkers of renal injury. *Journal of Applied Toxicology*, 32(6):417–428, 2012.

[365] A. Szabo. *CorrBin: Nonparametrics with clustered binary and multinomial data*, 2013. R package version 1.4.

[366] A. C. Tamhane and L. A. Hothorn. A multiple comparison procedure for three- and four-armed controlled clinical trials by M. A. Proschan in Statistics in Medicine 1999; 18 : 787-798. *Statistics in Medicine*, 20(2):317–318, 2001.

[367] M. C. Tamhane and B. R. Logan. A superiority-equivalence approach to one-sided tests on multiple endpoints in clinical trials. *Biometrika*, 91(3):715–727, September 2004.

[368] M. L. Tang, H. K. T. Ng, J. H. Guo, W. Chan, and B. P. S. Chan. Exact Cochran-Armitage trend tests: comparisons under different models. *Journal of Statistical Computation and Simulation*, 76(10):847–859, October 2006.

[369] R. E. Tarone. Tests for trend in life table analysis. *Biometrika*, 62(3):679–682, 1975.

[370] R.E. Tarone. The use of historical control information in testing for a trend in Poisson means. *Biometrics*, 38(2):457–462, 1982.

[371] P. Tattar. *gpk: 100 Data Sets for Statistics Education*, 2013. R package version 1.0.

[372] G.B. A Teuns, H. Geys, S.M. A Geuens, P. Stinissen, and T.F. Meert. Abuse liability assessment in preclinical drug development: Predictivity of a translational approach for abuse liability testing using methylphenidate in four standardized preclinical study models. *Journal of Pharmacological and Toxicological Methods*, 70(3):295–309, 2014.

[373] Terry Therneau. *survival: Survival analysis, including penalised likelihood.*, 2011. R package version 2.36-9, <http://CRAN.R-project.org/package=survival>.

[374] T.M. Therneau. *coxme: Mixed Effects Cox Models*, 2015. R package version 2.2-4.

[375] T.M. Therneau, P.M. Grambsch, and V.S. Pankratz. Penalized survival models and frailty. *Journal of Computational and Graphical Statistics*, 12(1):156–175, 2003.

[376] F. D. Toledo, L. M. Perez, C. L. Basiglio, J. E. Ochoa, E. J. S. Pozzi, and M. G. Roma. The ca2+-calmodulin-ca2+/calmodulin-dependent protein kinase ii signaling pathway is involved in oxidative stress-induced mitochondrial permeability transition and apoptosis in isolated rat hepatocytes. *Archives of Toxicology*, 88(9):1695–1709, 2014.

[377] Y. L. Tong. On partitioning a set of normal populations by their locations with respect to a control. *Annals of Mathematical Statistics*, 40(4):1300–1324, 1969.

[378] J. F. Troendle. A bootstrap test of stochastic equality of two populations - comment. *American Statistician*, 59(3):279–279, 2005.

[379] K.T. Tsai. Robust Williams trend test. *Communications in Statistics -Theory and Methods*, 29(5-6):1327–1346, 2000.

[380] J. W. Tukey, J. L. Ciminera, and J. F. Heyse. Testing the statistical certainty of a response to increasing doses of a drug. *Biometrics*, 41(1):295–301, 1985.

[381] F. Uibel, A. Muehleisen, C. Kohle, M. Weimer, T. C. Stummann, S. Bremer, and M. Schwarz. Reproglo: A new stem cell-based reporter assay aimed to predict embryotoxic potential of drugs and chemicals. *Reproductive Toxicology*, 30(1):103–112, 2010.

[382] L. N. Vandenberg. Non-monotonic dose responses in studies of endocrine disrupting chemicals: Bisphenol a as a case study. *Dose-response*, 12(2):259–276, 2014.

[383] P. Vasseur and C. Lasne. OECD Detailed Review Paper (DRP) number 31 on "Cell Transformation Assays for Detection of Chemical Carcinogens": Main results and conclusions. *Mutation Research-genetic Toxicology and Environmental Mutagenesis*, 744(1):8–11, 2012.

[384] W. N. Venables and B. D. Ripley. *Modern Applied Statistics with S*. Springer, New York, fourth edition, 2002. ISBN 0-387-95457-0.

[385] P. E. Verde, L. A. Geracitano, L. L. Amado, C. E. Rosa, A. Bianchini, and J. M. Monserrat. Application of public-domain statistical analysis software for evaluation and comparison of comet assay data. *Mutation Research-Genetic Toxicology and Environmental Mutagenesis*, 604(1-2):71–82, 2006.

[386] W. J. Waddell. History of dose response. *Journal of Toxicological Sciences*, 35(1):1–8, February 2010.

[387] T. Waldmann, E. Rempel, N. V. Balmer, A. Konig, R. Kolde, J. A. Gaspar, M. Henry, J. Hescheler, A. Sachinidis, J. Rahnenfuhrer, J. G. Hengstler, and M. Leist. Design principles of concentration-dependent transcriptome deviations in drug-exposed differentiating stem cells. *Chemical Research in Toxicology*, 27(3):408–420, 2014.

[388] D. I. Warton and F. K. C. Hui. The arcsine is asinine: The analysis of proportions in ecology. *Ecology*, 92(1):3–10, 2011.

[389] M. Weimer, X. Q. Jiang, O. Ponta, S. Stanzel, A. Freyberger, and A. Kopp-Schneider. The impact of data transformations on concentration-response modeling. *Toxicology Letters*, 213(2):292–298, 2012.

[390] B. West, K. Welch, and A. Galecki. *Linear Mixed Models: A Practical Guide Using Statistical Software*. Chapman Hall / CRC Press, first edition, 2006. ISBN 1584884800.

[391] B. T. West and A. T. Galecki. An overview of current software procedures for fitting linear mixed models. *American Statistician*, 65(4):274–282, 2011.

[392] P. Westfall. Proc multtest: Example 58.4 Fisher test with permutation resampling. Technical report, SAS Inc., 2014.

[393] P. H. Westfall and S. S. Young. P-value adjustments for multiple tests in multivariate binomial models. *Journal of the American Statistical Association*, 84(407):780–786, 1989.

[394] H. I. Weston, M. E. Sobolewski, J. L. Allen, D. Weston, K. Conrad, S. Pelkowski, G. E. Watson, G. Zareba, and D. A. Cory-Slechta. Sex-dependent and non-monotonic enhancement and unmasking of methylmercury neurotoxicity by prenatal stress. *Neurotoxicology*, 41:123–140, 2014.

[395] G. C. White and R. E. Bennetts. Analysis of frequency count data using the negative binomial distribution. *Ecology*, 77(8):2549–2557, 1996.

[396] H. Wickham. The split-apply-combine strategy for data analysis. *Journal of Statistical Software*, 40(1):1–29, 2011.

[397] H. Wickham and P. Hadley. Reshaping data with the reshape package. *Journal of Statistical Software*, 21(12), 2007.

[398] Hadley Wickham. *ggplot2: elegant graphics for data analysis*. Springer New York, 2009.

[399] S. J. Wiklund and E. Agurell. Aspects of design and statistical analysis in the comet assay. *Mutagenesis*, 18(2):167–175, 2003.

[400] D.A. Williams. A test for differences between treatment means when several dose levels are compared with a zero dose control. *Biometrics*, 27(1):103–117, 1971.

[401] D.A. Williams. The comparison of several dose levels with a zero dose control. *Biometrics*, 28(2):519–531, 1972.

[402] J. B. Wilson. Priorities in statistics, the sensitive feet of elephants, and don't transform data. *Folia Geobotanica*, 42(2):161–167, 2007.

[403] M. J. Wolfsegger, G. Gutjahr, W. Engl, and T. Jaki. A hybrid method to estimate the minimum effective dose for monotone and non-monotone dose-response relationships. *Biometrics*, 70(1):103–109, 2014.

[404] M. J. Wolfsegger and T. Jaki. Assessing systemic drug exposure in repeated dose toxicity studies in the case of complete and incomplete sampling. *Biometrical Journal*, 51(6):1017–1029, 2009.

[405] M. J. Wolfsegger and T. Jaki. Non-compartmental estimation of pharmacokinetic parameters in serial sampling designs. *Journal of Pharmacokinetics and Pharmacodynamics*, 36(5):479–494, 2009.

[406] M. J. Wolfsegger, T. Jaki, B. Dietrich, J. A. Kunzler, and K. Barker. A note on statistical analysis of organ weights in non-clinical toxicological studies. *Toxicology and Applied Pharmacology*, 240(1):117–122, 2009.

[407] G. H. Woo, M. Shibutani, T. Ichiki, M. Hamamura, K. Y. Lee, K. Inoue, and M. Hirose. A repeated 28-day oral dose toxicity study of nonylphenol in rats, based on the 'enhanced OECD test guideline 407' for screening of endocrine-disrupting chemicals. *Archives Of Toxicology*, 81(2):77–88, 2007.

[408] B. L. Wu and A. R. de Leon. Gaussian copula mixed models for clustered mixed outcomes, with application in developmental toxicology. *Journal of Agricultural Biological and Environmental Statistics*, 19(1):39–56, 2014.

[409] Y. Xie. *Dynamic Documents with R and knitr*. Chapman and Hall/CRC- The R Series, 2015.

[410] E. Yamamoto and T. Yanagimoto. Statistical-methods for the beta-binomial model in teratology. *Environmental Health Perspectives*, 102:25–31, 1994.

[411] T. Yanagawa and Y. Kikuchi. Statistical issues on the determination of the no-observed-adverse-effect levels in toxicology. *Environmetrics*, 12(4):319–325, 2001.

[412] Thomas W. Yee. The VGAM package for categorical data analysis. *Journal of Statistical Software*, 32(10):1–34, 2010.

[413] Thomas W. Yee. *VGAM: Vector Generalized Linear and Additive Models*, 2014. R package version 0.9-5.

[414] M. Yokohira, K. Hosokawa, K. Yamakawa, N. Hashimoto, S. Suzuki, Y. Matsuda, K. Saoo, T. Kuno, and K. Imaida. A 90-day toxicity study of l-asparagine, a food additive, in f344 rats. *Food and Chemical Toxicology*, 46(7):2568–2572, 2008.

[415] A. Zeileis. Object-oriented computation of sandwich estimators. *Journal of Statistical Software*, 16(9):1–16, 2006.

[416] A. Zeileis, C. Kleiber, and Simon Jackman. Regression models for count data in R. *Journal of Statistical Software*, 27(8):8, 2008.

[417] G. Zheng. Analysis of ordered categorical data: Two score-independent approaches. *Biometrics*, 64(4):1276–1279, 2008.

[418] D. W. Zimmerman. Type I error probabilities df the Wilcoxon-Mann-Whitney test and student t test altered by heterogeneous variances and equal sample sizes. *Perceptual And Motor Skills*, 88(2):556–558, 1999.

[419] D. W. Zimmerman. A note on preliminary tests of equality of variances. *British Journal of Mathematical & Statistical Psychology*, 57:173–181, 2004.

[420] D. W. Zimmerman and B. D. Zumbo. Rank transformations and the power of the student t-test and welch t-test for nonnormal populations with unequal variances. *Canadian Journal of Experimental Psychology-Revue Canadienne De Psychologie Experimentale*, 47(3):523–539, 1993.

[421] A. Zuur, E.N. Ieno, N. Walker, A.A. Saveliev, and G.M. Smith. *Mixed Effects Models and Extensions in Ecology with R (Statistics for Biology and Health)*. Springer, 2009 edition, 3 2009.

Index

Milton Keynes UK
Ingram Content Group UK Ltd.
UKHW051934141024
449569UK00027B/1481